PROFITS OF DEATH

An Insider Exposes
the Death Care Industries

Darryl J. Roberts

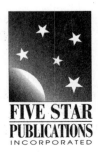

FIVE STAR
PUBLICATIONS
INCORPORATED

Published 1997 by Five Star Publications, Incorporated
Chandler, Arizona
Printed in the United States of America

Five Star Publications, Incorporated
P.O. Box 6698
Chandler, AZ 85246-6698
e-mail:info@fivestarsupport.com
http://www.fivestarsupport.com

Library of Congress Cataloging-in-Publication Data

Profits of Death:
    An Insider Exposes the Death Care Industries
        p.   cm.
    Includes index.
    ISBN: 1-877749-21-4
    1. Undertakers and undertaking--United States.
    2. Undertakers and undertaking--Social aspects--
        United States.
    3. Funeral rites and ceremonies--United States.
    4. Consumer education--United States.
I. Title.
Roberts, Darryl J., 1944-
HD9999.U53U572   1997
363.7'5'0973--dc21   96-53657
                                                      CIP

Publishing Consultant: Linda F. Radke
Editorial Consultant: Paul M. Howey
Cover Design: Lynlie Hermann
Typesetting & Layout: Toni Smith

Table of Contents

Table of Contents

Table of Contents

Table of Contents

Foreword

All funeral and cemetery practitioners know the deceptive methods used by many of their counterparts. Most are aware of the all-out legislative lobbying efforts of their respective industries. Few insiders, however, have tried to effect reform by publicizing the abuses. Mr. Roberts does just that, providing the kind of book the public needs–a book that hundreds of other death care professionals could have written over the years but did not. Despite the serious subject matter, spots of humor lighten and enliven the book throughout.

Families–especially those with modest and low incomes, many of the eldery, and persons who want simple arrangements–need to know how to obtain the lowest prices for various types of dispositions. Mr. Roberts is to be complimented for his straightforward explanation of so much of the funeral process and industry that people have wondered about and need to understand. Consumers, religious leaders, and the media will all benefit from his information about sales methods, casket wholesale costs and markups, embalming, cremation, and suggestions about how to arrange for more economical funeral and burial.

This book will help protect from financial harm many who have picked up misconceptions and poor "consumer advice" from the funeral and cemetery industries, their national association offices, the media, and even some financial magazines.

Rev. Henry Wasielewski

Editor's Note: Rev. Wasielewski, a priest of the Catholic Diocese of Phoenix, was a member of a group of laypersons and clergy from various denominations that founded the Interfaith Funeral Information Committee (IFIC) in 1982. The IFIC has conducted thousands of hours of research and provided assistance to many media investigations of the funeral and cemetery industries. He has appeared on several network television shows in the U.S. including ABC-TV's "Home," NBC-TV's "Today" and "Dateline," and CNBC-TV's "Steals and Deals" and in documentaries by BBC-TV in England. He is the recipient of a special Social Justice Award presented by the Catholic Diocese of Phoenix in 1991 for his work among farm workers and prisoners and for his work in exposing funeral industry abuses. You can obtain information about current funeral prices by contacting the IFIC by calling (602) 253-6814 or by visiting the organization's website in the Internet (www.xroads.com/~funerals).

Introduction

She was sitting right there in the front row and she flipped me off! I was delivering a speech promoting *"cooperation* between the funeral and cemetery industries" at a West Virginia funeral business conference. The woman, who was the wife of a funeral director, apparently disagreed with what she was hearing.

I've been in and around the funeral and cemetery businesses nearly all my life. Granted, it was probably different from the way you were raised; but for me, and others like me, it was a perfectly normal life. Historically, funeral homes and cemeteries have been family-run businesses, passed down from one generation to the next.

I began working summers at my father's cemetery when I was 12. One of my first jobs was helping with the construction of a mausoleum. The workers needed someone to go inside each of the 100 crypts and clean out the excess concrete that had dropped on the floors. As I was the smallest member of the work crew, I was chosen to chisel out the concrete and then sweep out each of the crypts. During those first few years, I also handled the mowing and trimming duties around the cemetery.

When I was 15, I "graduated" to digging graves. We were yet to buy our first backhoe, so the graves were all dug by hand with shovels. My father would drop me off at the cemetery each morning and I would take the bus home in the afternoon. I had this job June through August during my high school years. The summer following my freshman year at college, I began selling cemetery lots. After that, I stayed in school year-round so I wouldn't have to sell so much!

After I graduated from college in 1967, my father asked me to manage a cemetery he had purchased in Richlands, Virginia, where he had also acquired a funeral home. That fall, I had the privilege (okay, even *I* didn't consider it a privilege!) of witnessing my first embalming. I managed the cemetery and coordinated the activities of the funeral home for the next two years. In late 1969, I became business manager for our family-owned business of cemeteries and funeral homes. After my father's death in 1980, I was named president of the corporation and ran the company until I sold it in the fall of 1994.

I know from experience that the funeral and cemetery operations—the death merchants, if you will—are a potent marketing and political force. They have, over the years, succeeded in creating an exclusionary business atmosphere in which they strictly limit competition and control pricing. Add in the proclivity of too many industry practitioners for preying on the emotionally vulnerable and you have what I consider to be an intolerable situation.

Please understand that there are conscientious operators in the funeral and cemetery industries as there are in any field. My only purpose is to expose those who appear to profit without regard to conscience and to provide consumers the knowledge that is necessary to make informed decisions.

The practitioners and lobbyists of the death merchant industries have long exhibited a "circle the wagons" mentality whenever someone has dared to speak critically of them. I fully expect, and welcome, their rebuttals of this book. The National Funeral Directors Association and the International Cemetery and Funeral Association have a long record of furnishing their members with what can only be described as propaganda with which to discredit anyone brazen enough to find fault with industry practices. In my particular case, I imagine that they will say, "Who is he to criticize? He participated in the same questionable sales practices about which he is now so publicly critical." Of that, I must admit I am guilty. They will probably add that I made a great deal of money from my funeral home and cemetery operations. Of that, too, I am fortunately "guilty." And, no doubt, they will criticize me by asking, "If he felt so strongly, why was he not a greater voice for reform while he was still in the business and, therefore, in a better position to effect change?" These are fair criticisms. In my partial defense, I did try to make some improvements. However, I must confess I did not do nearly enough. I cannot right that wrong by remaining silent.

I have no ulterior motives for writing this book. Its purpose is straightforward: to help educate. For only if the consuming public is informed and only if it is aware can it adequately protect itself from those who only see the profits of death. I hope this book helps.

Darryl J. Roberts

P.S. Oh, and about that funeral director's wife sitting in the front row? Her husband died and I bought her funeral home after which she was exceedingly cordial!

Prologue

We would not hold the ceremony at our funeral home because we were warned in advance that the parishioners would be handling poisonous snakes. Their use of live rattlesnakes in regular worship services was widely known throughout our small West Virginia community. In fact, this funeral was for the church leader who had been bitten by one of the rattlesnakes and died.

Although this was our first attempt at providing funeral services for one of their followers, we knew our proper role was not to judge. Discretion dictated, however, that we hold the funeral service outside our facilities. Therefore, we embalmed the body and then had everyone gather at their church. There was much chanting and dancing as they placed two live rattlers in the coffin. One crawled around the casket, in and out of the suit of the deceased, up the arm, and finally curled up next to his head. The other snake went to the foot of the casket.

The church elder finally closed the lid of the coffin at the conclusion of the service, trapping the snakes inside. We couldn't get our minds off the reptiles and what they might possibly be doing in there as we drove to the cemetery. We cautiously removed the coffin from the hearse and carried it to the grave site. We wondered among ourselves whether the snakes were to be released before the body was lowered into the grave. They were not, and they went to their grave along with their unwitting human host.

I include this story to illustrate that the funeral director's primary responsibility should be to understand and serve the needs and wishes of the consumer. The purpose of using the word "consumer" is to show that this is a business—there are providers and there are consumers, sellers, and buyers. It is a business that should be run like any other. It should provide its services and products on an honest, profitable yet competitive, basis. The fact that it does not has been the subject of several books, investigative reports by the media, and Congressional inquiries for years. But nothing has really changed. Why not? There is no single answer. Partly, it is because of the extraordinarily strong and naturally self-serving lobbying efforts of the funeral and cemetery industries. Partly, it is because the public—though temporarily outraged—has not mounted an organized effort to do anything about it. Partly, it is because of the subject itself: death. Death and the consequences of dealing with death and paying for death are most often ignored until one has no alternative. But by then, the death merchants have us right where they want us—vulnerable, emotional, susceptible, and with checkbooks in hand.

This book alone will not make a difference. But, in conjunction with all the other attempts to bring to light the abuses of the death industry, perhaps it will help. My purpose in writing this book is twofold: to demystify the whole business of funerals and burials and to inform the consumers as to their rightful choices. An informed public is a protected public.

1

Behind Closed Doors

A Close Look at Death and Embalming

"No American is prepared to attend his own funeral without the services of highly skilled cosmeticians. Part of the American dream, after all, is to live long and die young."
  Edgar Z. Friendenberg, *The Vanishing Adolescent* (1959)

AUTHOR'S NOTE: While what follows may appear to border on the macabre and sensationalistic, I believe it is important to understand what happens after someone dies and to know what happens behind the mortuary's closed doors. If you don't want to have this type of information, then I suggest you skip to the next chapter. Bear in mind, however, that much of the manipulative marketing strength of the death merchants is predicated on your having little or no knowledge of exactly what they do to earn their money. The death merchants would like to keep it that way.

I understand the pervasive and persuasive desire to believe that the bodies of our deceased loved ones undergo the embalming process in order to preserve their earthly appearance for all time. The truth, however, is that injecting the body with a formaldehyde solution retards the natural process of decomposition by only a few days.

The sole purpose of the embalming procedure is to present the body in the most pleasant way possible (not to mention, to further increase the profits of the funeral director). The funeral industry has long promoted the concept that embalming permits the viewing of the body and that viewing the body somehow permits friends and loved ones to be better able to accept the death and to say their fond farewells. One should note, however, that the ritual of embalming for viewing the dead is primarily an American phenomenon. While this practice has become accepted in the United States and Canada (and, to a lesser degree, Australia), it is rarely used in Europe. It has recently become more common in the United Kingdom; however, cosmetics are seldom applied to the deceased. Elsewhere throughout the world, we are looked upon with bewilderment and some disgust for our burial practices. Perhaps this fact is the greatest single testament to the marketing abilities of our funeral professionals. It becomes even more remarkable when you learn exactly what the embalming process entails.

You still with me? Good—then please read on.

Dust to Dust

Death is actually a series of processes, not a single event. Most people incorrectly believe that death occurs at the point when a person ceases to breathe and the heart no longer beats. This is technically known as *somatic death*, the person is irretrievably gone, but the death process is actually just beginning. In actuality, the cells of the body's tissues and organs die at varying rates over a period of the next several minutes. The brain cells are particularly susceptible to the lack of oxygen and are among the first to die, usually within the first three to seven minutes. The other organs soon follow.

One of the first things to occur after the heart stops beating is the body's drop in temperature, a process known as *algor mortis*. The temperature will continue to drop until the body reaches the same temperature as the air around it, usually in fewer than three hours. Normally within two days, however, the body temperature will begin to rise again due to the bacterial activity in the decomposing body. Bacteria, protozoa, and other organisms omnipresent in the living body begin to multiply, attacking first the intestines and the blood. The body's organs decompose at different, fairly predictable rates which enable coroners to estimate the time of death. Also, coroners can often establish the sex of the corpse because the uterus and the prostate gland are among the last organs to completely decompose (these organs are frequently nearly intact a full year after death). Granted, death is not a pretty picture, but it is among the most natural of life's events.

The five stages of decomposition are fairly standard, although the length of each is dependent on a variety of factors including the location of the body and the surrounding temperature and climate.

During the **initial stage**, also known as the "fresh stage," the flesh appears normal though decomposition of the internal organs has already begun. The skin pales as the blood begins, through force of gravity, to settle in the parts of the body lowest to the ground. *Livor mortis* is the term used to describe the purplish discoloration of the skin surrounding the lower blood vessels.

The **putrefaction stage**, also known as the "bloat stage," follows, during which the body appears distended due to the internal gases created by the decomposition, and there is usually a distinct odor of decay. An initial indication of putrefaction is a greenish color in the abdominal skin that then advances to the chest and thighs. Both the odor and the discoloration result from the sulfurous gas in the intestines and from the progressive disintegration of the red blood cells. The gas can cause the tongue and eyes to protrude. A bloody discharge frequently oozes from the mouth and nose.

The **black putrefaction stage,** also known as the "advanced decay stage," follows. The flesh appears almost liquid in texture, the abdominal cavity collapses, and the odor of decaying flesh is quite apparent. By now, most of the skin is discolored and the uppermost layers will come off in sheets if handled too roughly (also known as "skin slip"). At this point, the bloated internal organs start to rupture and release their liquids. The gas that creates the bloating can force the intestines outside the body through the vagina and anus.

The body then begins to dry out during what is called the **butyric stage,** also known as the "fermentation stage." Bits of flesh remain, and there may be a cheese-like smell and mold on the abdominal area. Finally, **dry decay,** also known as the "skeletal stage," is when the corpse is almost completely dry and little, if any, flesh remains.

Depending upon environmental conditions, the first three stages of death can be rather swift and are often accompanied by the presence of maggots. Following the third stage, the mass of the corpse decreases noticeably due largely to the work of the maggots and to the loss, through seepage, of body fluids. The final two stages of decomposition can be rather protracted, again depending upon the surrounding conditions such as temperature, humidity, etc.

Rigor Mortis (...or Why They Call Them "Stiffs")

As long as a person is alive, the muscles of the body work both aerobically and anaerobically (i.e., with and without oxygen). Lactic acid is the by-product of anaerobic activity and, in the living person, is broken down through the intake of oxygen. When the lungs stop functioning, the cells of the muscles can only operate anaerobically and the lactic acid builds up. Over a short period of time, this lactic acid buildup turns to a gelatinous consistency that results in a stiffening of the body.

When a person dies, the muscles of the body relax momentarily ("primary flaccidity"), but rigor mortis begins soon afterward, starting first in the eyelids, neck, and jaw muscles. Over the next four- to six-hour period (more quickly in colder weather and if the person had experienced strenuous physical exertion before death), rigor mortis extends to the body's other muscles, including those of the internal organs. Generally, rigor mortis continues until the decomposition of the body is well under way, usually within one to three days. At

15

that point, the muscles once again relax ("secondary flaccidity").

Funeral directors must be prepared to handle bodies in all conditions (e.g., bodies in various stages of decomposition, accident victims, decapitations, drowning victims, etc.). Realizing all that, aren't you grateful that at least *some* people are willing to be undertakers? And just what is it that morticians do to the body after it is delivered to their funeral home?

A Brief History of Embalming

The word *embalm*, in the beginning, literally meant to place balm—a mixture of tree or pine sap and aromatic spices—in the body after removing the internal organs and then allowing the body to dry out. Modern embalming replaces the blood and other fluids of the body with solutions designed to retard decomposition. Embalming, according to a funeral director's handbook, "is the art of disinfecting dead bodies and thereby slowing the process of decomposition." In other words, the handbook admits that the decomposition of the body is merely "slowed" rather than prevented—a major distinction often obscured by funeral directors when they sell surviving family members on the idea of embalming.

The issue of disinfection is another matter of some continuing contention (and I fully expect that funeral directors will attempt to refute what I am about to say). Undertakers, certainly in their lobbying efforts with state legislatures and Congress, have long contended that they play a vital role in protecting the public health through their recommended embalming and burial procedures. They have maintained, and the consuming public and governmental regulatory bodies have largely accepted, that embalming decontaminates the corpse rendering it incapable of spreading infection to the living. Donald E. Douthit, Director of Research at the Cincinnati College of Mortuary Science, writes: "Today, the licensed funeral service professional is truly an extension of the public health service. It is the moral, ethical, and legal duty of each licensed funeral director and embalmer to protect the welfare of the public by handling the deceased in a manner prescribed in guidelines to protect the public as well as themselves from potential health threats." The truth is, of course, that a corpse represents practically no infectious risk, especially when compared to a living person. A corpse no longer breathes, excretes, or perspires—the primary means by which contagious diseases are spread; and a body dead of a noncommunicable disease presents virtually no threat at all. Lest someone attempt to contradict this premise by citing the historic plagues such as typhoid and cholera, it should be pointed out that even modern embalming processes are incapable of completely eliminating the organisms that cause these diseases.

Some funeral homes have attempted to charge more for embalming a body that suffered from an infectious disease prior to death. As embalmers are required by law to treat all bodies the same, it is a violation of the Americans with Disabilities Act (ADA) to tack on an additional charge for those cases involving infectious diseases. Still, some funeral homes have refused to embalm bodies of AIDS victims. This, too, is illegal. The ADA "requires funeral homes to provide their services on a non-discriminatory basis to persons who have AIDS..."

17

Thomas H. Holmes is most frequently cited as the father of modern embalming. Holmes got his start, and his considerable wealth, embalming soldiers killed in the Civil War. He claimed to have embalmed more than 4,000 bodies in just four years, focusing on those of officers whose families he knew were able to pay his $100 charge. Using various mixtures (he never revealed the exact formulae) of arsenic and zinc chloride, Holmes claimed that those he embalmed would be preserved forever.

As recently as the late 1800s, though, undertakers preserved bodies prior to burial by cooling them with ice. At most, they would apply embalming solutions to the skin of the corpses. They lacked the tools and knowledge to effectively inject the solutions into the bodies (early attempts at injection embalming frequently left the body hard and stone-like). As the science of medicine and the knowledge of the human body progressed, the "art" of embalming tagged along, appropriating some of that new information and the tools developed to aid the living. What follows are the procedures used in a typical modern embalming.

A "How-To" Manual of Embalming

WARNING! **Embalmers are paid professionals. Please! Do *not* attempt these procedures at home.**

Into the early 1950s, embalming was routinely done in the home of the deceased, often with family members present. The undertaker would bring his embalming table and tools and would flush the fluids from the body down the drain. Now, of course, the procedure is done behind the closed doors of the mortuary and the average person's knowledge of what goes on has greatly diminished.

The embalming room—or the preparation room, as funeral directors prefer to call it—often has a separate ventilation system to remove odors so as not to commingle them with the air circulating throughout the rest of the funeral home. The embalmer usually dons a surgical apron or full-body surgical suit, latex gloves, and protective goggles. The body is then laid out on a stainless steel or porcelain table similar to those used for autopsies (a mechanical body lift is frequently used to place the body on the table). Next, the clothing is removed from the corpse and any personal possessions are recorded. Items of jewelry that are removed are replaced on the body after it is embalmed, or they are given to the family.

The cadaver is then washed with a combination germicide-insecticide. In addition to cleaning the body, the solution also kills any maggots and other insects that might be present and it helps eliminate any odors that may be emanating from the body. The embalmer then uses the solution to swab the insides of the mouth and nose.

Frequently, fluid from the stomach and lungs (descriptively referred to as "purge" by embalmers) is ejected through the mouth and nose. Therefore, it is sometimes necessary to turn the body over in order to permit the fluids to drain out and, if needed, to be suctioned out. To prevent a recurrence of purge, the trachea and esophagus are sometimes cut and tied off when the neck is opened during the actual embalming process.

Before positioning the body for embalming, it may be necessary to massage and bend the arms and legs to relieve rigor mortis. If the limbs are deformed—perhaps through arthritis, disease, or birth defects—the embalmer may slice through the tendons and muscles in order to be able to place the limbs in a more natural pose.

The body is then washed again, this time with a combination of warm soapy water and disinfectant bleach to kill any remaining bacteria, and then towel dried. Any blood on the body or hair is washed away and the fingernails are cleaned and manicured.

At this point, the nose is aligned by inserting wads of cotton. The eyes are closed using eyecaps, round plastic devices that are covered with knobs designed to grip the inside of the eyelids and keep them closed. Much care is taken to position the eyelids in a manner that appears to be the most relaxed, neither pained nor squinting; the preferred position being with the upper lid closed two-thirds of the way and the lower lid the other third, just touching each other and not overlapping. The eyelids are sometimes glued together to prevent them from opening (not a comforting sight when that occurs!).

The throat is then packed with cotton or gauze and a mouth former, similar to the eyecaps, is inserted to prevent the mouth and cheeks from appearing sunken and to keep the lips together (some embalmers inject a mastic substance into the mouth to help shape the cheeks). The next implement used is a piece of wire with a fishhook-like barb at each end. The embalmer imbeds one barb in the upper gum just above the teeth line and the other barb in the lower. The wire is then simply twisted to close the mouth. As with the eyelids, great care is taken to shape the lips into the most favorable and natural-looking expression possible, neither snarling nor too smiling in appearance. To keep the lips together, they, too, may be glued shut. The anus and vagina are then packed with pieces of gauze or cotton that are soaked in an embalming fluid and a close-fitting plastic undergarment may be placed on the body—all to contain any seepage of fluids. At this point, a massage cream is worked into the face and hands. The body is now ready for the actual embalming process to begin.

One or more of the following methods are utilized: *arterial embalming*, in which the embalming fluids are injected into the body's blood vessels; *cavity embalming*, in which the torso is injected with the fluids; *hypodermic* or *syringe embalming*, in which the formaldehyde solution is injected under the skin; and *surface embalming*, in which the embalming fluids are applied on the outside of the body. In most modern embalmings, the arterial and cavity methods are used together, and the hypodermic or syringe methods are used as needed to complete the embalming in areas not reached by the other methods. The surface procedure is used primarily on infants and on body parts that may be injured or mangled.

There are eight major points of entry for arterial embalming: the left and right carotid arteries located on either side of the neck, the left and right femoral arteries located in the inside of the upper thighs, the left and right axillary arteries located in the upper shoulders, and the left and right iliac arteries located between the hip bones and the pubic bone. The veins corresponding to the arteries chosen are used to drain the blood. The condition of the body and its arterial and vasculatory systems will determine how many points of injection will be required.

For efficiency and economy, as few points as possible are used—only one if possible. The selection is normally made from four points (the right and/or left carotid artery, the right axillary artery, and/or the right femoral artery). The body of an obese person, for example, may require more injection points in order for the fluids to adequately reach all of the extremities. Other determining factors would be if the body had been autopsied or if there had been organ donation.

Once the embalmer has selected the artery, an incision is made. The flesh is folded back and the artery and corresponding vein are pulled out and held above the surface of the skin to permit the insertion of the injection and blood drainage instruments known as cannulae.

The embalming fluid—a mixture of water and about 40% formaldehyde and other additives depending upon the condition of the corpse—is pumped under pressure into the body. Normally, three or four gallons of the embalming fluid are pumped into the chosen arteries (nearly twice that amount is used in embalming cadavers for anatomical dissection, explaining why these bodies are able to last as long as they do and why their skin appears dark and leathery), forcing the blood out through the drainage tubes in the veins. The pump pulses the fluid through the body in order to dislodge any blood clots that might be present. The blood exiting the body is channeled through gutters in the embalming table to buckets or, in some instances, directly into the sewer system. While it is impossible to remove all of the blood, it is important to remove as much as possible in order to minimize discoloration of the skin.

Once the injections are completed, the arteries and vessels that were used are tied off and the incisions made to access them are sutured shut. The embalmer then repeatedly thrusts a long, sharp, hollow metal instrument, known as a *trocar*, into the abdominal cavity in several different directions to pierce the internal organs. The trocar is connected to an aspirator pump and is used to suck out the fluids and gas from the stomach, bladder, large intestines, and lungs. Once these have been removed, the pump is reversed and the trocar is then used to inject an embalming preservative into the abdomen and chest and, if the arterial process was not totally successful, into the penis and scrotum. The trocar can also be inserted into the skull through the nose to remove gas and fluids and then used to inject cavity embalming fluid through the same opening.

Holes caused by the trocar are then either sutured shut or, as is the more common practice today, closed by means of plastic trocar buttons that are inserted into the openings.

Once the embalming solution has been injected into the body, the muscles begin to stiffen again and become hard within eight to twelve hours. Once this occurs, the limbs can no longer be adjusted.

The true artistry of the embalmer may be called upon if restoration is necessary. Accident victims, autopsied corpses, organ donors, and others may require the embalmer to turn sculptor, molding wax replacement ears, noses, lips, hands, etc., to render the body complete. Sometimes, as in the cases of some amputations or decapitations, the embalmer may sew the appendage or head back onto the body, covering the stitches with makeup or clothing, such as a high collar or longer sleeves.

The embalming procedure is now complete. The body is again washed and dried, dressed, and ready for final placement. The head is slightly raised and tilted to the right (the commonly preferred angle for viewing) the arms are folded, and the hands placed across the chest. To keep them from separating, the fingers are glued together. Then either the embalmer (or, as is often the case, a professional hair stylist) will wash and set the hair. Then, if needed, the face is shaved, and any facial hair and distracting blemishes are either removed or covered up. Cosmetics are applied to the face, neck, and hands in an effort to render a more a "life-like" appearance to the corpse. The body is now ready to be placed into the casket (or, in the argot of funeral directors, *casketed*).

YOU SAY TO-MAY-TO
AND I SAY TO-MAW-TO

The sanitizing of the death merchants' language is a never-ending challenge to its practitioners. Through the euphemistic manipulation of words, these folks believe they are creating an environment in which the process of dealing with death (and the process of parting consumers from their cash) will become easier. All professions develop their own lingo over time, sometimes for the purpose of being exclusionary and sometimes for the purpose of trying to elevate their profession in the eyes of the public. Regardless of how you view it, language "cleansing" is a subtle art of seduction.

WHAT IT IS (or *used* to be called)	WHAT *THEY* CALL IT
ashes	cremains
body	deceased or decedent (also commonly referred to by name as Mr., Mrs., Miss, or Ms. _____)
burial of ashes	inurnment
burial plot salesperson	family service counselor
bury	inter
casket showroom	display room
cemetery operator	cemeterian
coffin	casket
cost of the casket and burial	investment in the service
dead	expired
embalming	creating a "memory picture"
embalming room	preparation room
embalming schools	colleges of mortuary science
funeral	service
funeral job	call
graveyard	cemetery or memorial gardens
putting the body in the casket	casketing
putting the casket in a mausoleum	immuring
removing a body	transferring
retort	cremation chamber
undertaker or mortician	funeral director

Requirements and Costs of Embalming

Through patently misleading marketing ploys, the funeral industry long led people to believe that embalming was a legal requirement, even in the case of cremations. The Federal Trade Commission, in its Funeral Rule issued in 1984, prohibited funeral directors from embalming for a fee unless "state or local law requires embalming" or "prior approval for embalming" has been obtained from the family.

Still the misrepresentation persists. Mr. Douthit of the Cincinnati College of Mortuary Science writes, "For example, embalming may be required as a condition of public viewing, known as calling hours or visitation which are predicated (sic) by the funeral home to ensure the safety of the public paying their respects, as well as protecting the employees' welfare who have contact with the deceased." The truth is, while practicality may dictate the need for embalming if there is to be a viewing, the law does not. Further, when the law does require embalming, it is seldom for public health reasons but more to minimize the unpleasant odors of an unembalmed person awaiting burial. Many states require that bodies be embalmed if burial is not going to occur within a certain number of days. Other states do not require embalming if the body is refrigerated and taken from the cooler for no more than two or three hours in order to have a viewing, or if there is a closed-casket service. Normally, embalming is required only if the body is to be shipped across state or international boundaries.

There is no religious "requirement" to embalm. It is more a practice of theological tolerance than an endorsement of the process. The majority of the embalmings in the United States today are of those of the Christian faith, although in earlier times, embalming was prohibited by the Christian hierarchy. Most other religions either discourage or actually prohibit the embalming of their dead.

EERIE...BUT TRUE

As hopefully demonstrated by the snake handler funeral that I recounted in the introduction to this book, I always encouraged our funeral directors to meet the customer's wishes whenever possible.

We had a customer, a wealthy gentleman who, as of the writing of this book, is still well and quite alive. As part of his pre-need arrangements, he directed our funeral home to mummify his body to the greatest extent modern technology will allow and place him in a hermetically sealed casket with a glass lid. He has bequeathed rather significant sums of money to various relatives on one condition: within two years of his death, they are to come to our establishment and view his body.

Interestingly, the funeral home will have to keep this fellow lying around in the garage for a couple of years waiting for his kinfolk to come and see him. Once they have seen his body and signed the necessary paperwork, they will be entitled to their share of his estate.

<u>Ours is not to question why....ours is but to mummify</u>!

Funeral directors are preoccupied with promoting the professionalism of their vocation. Granted, learning how to properly embalm does require knowledge of the body's vascular system, but I don't believe that knowing how to embalm necessarily connotes any special level of professionalism.

Actually, due to the ever-increasing complexity of today's automobiles with all their new computers and safety devices, a mechanic is more deserving of professional respect. Consider for a moment that mechanic who must be current in knowledge of perhaps twenty or thirty years' worth of cars, even if they are all of the same make. Humans come in all shapes and sizes, but underneath it all our vascular systems are remarkably similar year in and year out. In a thinly disguised move to "professionalize" the funeral profession, aspiring morticians no longer attend a school of embalming. No. Now they go to a *college of mortuary science.* Same school, faculty, and courses as before—just a fancier, presumably more prestigious, title. For the record, beginning embalmers earn an average of $6.50 per hour.

Every state requires their funeral directors to be licensed, and some states require an additional embalming license. Funeral directors, however, do not have to be embalmers and embalmers do not need to be funeral directors. Though in reality, most funeral directors are embalmers. Hey, why pay out just slightly more than minimum wage plus benefits to someone else? To maintain their licenses, funeral directors and embalmers in several states must fulfill continuing education requirements set forth by the funeral industry itself (23 states—including California, Michigan, New York, and Pennsylvania, with their nearly 20,000 funeral directors and embalmers—don't require any continuing education whatsoever to maintain their licenses). In some states, the continuing education requirement is met simply by going to one trade meeting every other year.

Licensing and meaningless continuing education requirements are, in my opionion, just another ploy by the industry to limit competition. The funeral director sells caskets and vaults. Does the electronics superstore salesperson have to be licensed to sell computers or television sets that are far more complex than a wood or concrete box? Anyway, off my soapbox and back to the embalming at hand.

For the embalmer's work, which may take from two to eight hours to complete, the charge in 1991, according to the National Funeral Directors Association's *Survey of Funeral Operations*, was $226.23. Other charges, for such things as cosmetology and hair styling, averaged $90.71, for a total embalming bill of $316.94. In my experience, embalming normally ran between $200 and $500, occasionally higher depending upon the circumstances (e.g., cause of death, size of the deceased, amount of decomposition, etc.). There is certainly some profit built into these charges, especially after learning how much embalmers earn for their efforts.

I don't imagine many of you, after reading this chapter, are going to begrudge embalmers their salary, nor do I envision you opting for a career change!

2

The Fashion Merchandise of Funerals

The "Stuff" They'll Try to Sell You

"It makes small difference to the dead, if they are buried in the tokens of luxury. All this is an empty glorification left for those who live."
Euripedes, *The Trojan Women* (415 B.C.)

The array of accoutrements available to the consumer through the funeral home is wide (from caskets to vaults to burial clothes to flowers to thank-you cards, and more). Funeral directors are more than happy—indeed, they are well-trained—to steer the emotionally distracted consumer through the dizzying variety of choices. The purpose of this chapter is to serve as a guide to making the best choices.

First, we'll discuss caskets and vaults. Let's get one thing straight—just as embalming forestalls only momentarily the natural process of decomposition, there is no casket nor grave vault that will keep out the elements for all time. All the advertising claims, sales pitches, implied warranties, and innuendoes to the contrary, there is nothing that can prevent the disintegration of the casket nor stem the flow of water into a vault. Yet, it's just such implied claims that persuade the consumer to frequently overspend in order to believe they are buying some kind of protection for the departed and so that the deceased will be "as comfortable as possible."

Caskets and Coffins

What is the difference between a casket and a coffin? Despite funeral directors' never-ending quest for euphemistic perfection, they are one and the same. In their drive to purge from our language the words and terms they feel detract from the marketability of their products and services, the funeral industry is wont to replace them with more pleasant-sounding words. The casket/coffin dispute is a case in point.

Most funeral directors will tell you that a coffin is a six-sided box, built roughly in the shape of the human body (narrow at the head, wider at the shoulders, and tapering along the legs), and is essentially relegated to funeral history. Clarence W. Miller, a self-proclaimed 35-year veteran of the funeral business, tells his readers in his *The Funeral Book* (1994, Robert D. Reed, Publishers): "Caskets are often mistakenly referred to as coffins. You cannot buy a coffin in the United States. They are not manufactured here except by private individuals. Coffins are made in other parts of the world. Technically, both do the same thing, but they are as different as a Volkswagen and a Rolls Royce. A coffin is a different shape. It has six sides, wide at the shoulders and narrow at the feet. This is the original coffin known as a burial container by the layman."

Mr. Miller challenges his readers to "Look it up in your dictionary." Being an obedient sort, I did just that—in four different dictionaries by four separate publishers. Each said that a casket was a box in which a corpse is buried. Each said the same thing about coffins, too. And no reference was made in any of them to a six-sided description-definition of coffins. I did, however, find one definition that explains the proclivity of funeral directors to prefer using the word "casket" instead of "coffin." That definition gives credence to Mr. Miller's statement that "they are as different as a Volkswagen and a Rolls Royce." In my hefty ten-pound edition of *Webster's New Twentieth Century Dictionary Unabridged,* I read the following definition of the word "casket": "A coffin, especially a costly one." Ahh, *costly*...that explains everything now!

If you have two identical boxes and you can sell the one called a "casket" for two to six times the amount you can get for the one called a "coffin," what would you do? You bet! You'd think like a funeral director. And you probably wouldn't stop there; and neither have the funeral directors nor the casket manufacturers.

A casket/coffin is a box in which to bury human remains. It is that and nothing more. But because consumers are persuaded that it is so much more, they are often seduced into paying extraordinary prices for that box. Caskets are big business and provide the highest profit margin to the funeral director of all the goods and services he or she provides. But, because the consumer has had little or no knowledge of the wholesale prices of caskets, the death merchants have been quite successful at getting away with charging as much as possible.

One Size (Nearly) Fits All

Caskets come in a myriad of designs and styles and are constructed of a variety of materials, from the simple pine box to the ornately elaborate bronze sarcophagus. Also, they come in quite a few different sizes. Beyond the obvious size differences for infants and children, there are different sizes available for adults, although most funeral homes do not routinely stock larger sizes.

Funeral directors are creative folks, though, and they can usually find ways to "make do" with what's in stock. What do they do? For a very tall individual, the funeral director may be able to bend the legs or may remove the shoes to make the body fit into the box. For an obese individual with a protruding belly, the funeral director may turn the body slightly to one side and may position the hands further down so the lid can be closed.

The Story behind the Coffin

Early in our country's history, coffins were often manufactured as a sideline for furniture makers. Many of these folks also began to serve as undertakers (the word "undertaker" literally meant an individual who would *undertake* to prepare a body for burial) as a means to make more money. It was several years before undertaking became a specialized field. Eventually, companies came into existence just to make coffins. Kenneth V. Iserson, M.D., in his book *Death to Dust* (1994, Galen Press, Ltd.) wrote that the coffin makers organized the National Burial Case Association to "set industry-wide prices—with a 40% price increase in 1881. This spurred undertakers to organize their trade, so they could control funeral prices and collectively bargain with manufacturers for funeral merchandise." Market control in this business got off to an early start! Given that background and combined with the ever-present need for increased profit, it is not at all surprising to understand the evolution of the pine box into a "masterpiece" of construction costing several thousand dollars.

Accessorizing Your Casket

Much goes into determining the price of a casket: material, finish, craftsmanship, hardware, lining, mattress, style (i.e., full couch, allowing viewing of the entire body; and half-couch, permitting viewing from the waist up). Let's examine these variables to better understand what is being presented to the consumer.

The mattress and pillow used in less expensive caskets are low-end quality and frequently filled with sawdust or wood shavings. The quality and construction of the bedding generally keeps pace with the overall increase in quality of the casket. The high-end caskets can even include an innerspring adjustable mattress! While such an amenity appears ludicrous, and rightly so, morticians claim it enables them to more easily and more properly display the body. The idea of an innerspring adjustable mattress for a dead person strikes me as truly absurd—it's just another way in which the funeral directors profit by fostering the image of "eternal rest."

Inexpensive materials—generally a manmade fabric such as rayon—are used to line caskets in the lower price ranges. In the higher priced caskets, the lining is luxuriously upholstered in a much more expensive material such as satin or velvet that is often sewn in intricate design patterns.

The hardware (i.e., the handles and hinges) chosen can also markedly affect the price, as can the addition of scenes displayed in the underside of the lid and other sculpted designs (e.g., praying hands, the Last Supper, flowers, etc.) that can be attached to the top of coffin. Bear in mind that the casket you purchase is yours to do with as you choose; no permission is required to add personal touches such as photographs, artwork, mementos, etc. You are not required to select from the options offered by the funeral director.

Casket Construction

Wood Caskets—At the lower end of the price spectrum of wood caskets are those made of a pressed particle board and covered with cloth. A step up from these are the plain pine caskets commonly used for the burial of orthodox Jews and constructed without any metal whatsoever (they're held together by wood dowels and glue in place of screws) and often without any interior lining. Particle board and pine caskets comprise less than 10% of all casket sales. The more expensive hardwood caskets (e.g., those made of oak, walnut, cherry, mahogany, etc.) are finished in a style comparable to the finest furniture. As the quality of the wood and the craftsmanship and accessories increase, the price also increases. Hardwood caskets account for about 15% of all casket sales.

EERIE...BUT TRUE

Occasionally, caskets can be rather poorly constructed. At one graveside service, the pallbearers were taking a body to the grave when the bottom literally fell out of the casket, dumping the poor deceased out on the ground in front of the somber gathering of family and friends. It's surprising this doesn't happen more often. What would cars be like if they were built to last for only two or three days?!

Steel Caskets—At the low-price end of metal caskets are those made of steel (steel caskets represent nearly three-fourths of all caskets sold). Steel is measured in gauges; most common for caskets are: 20-gauge, 18-gauge, and 16-gauge. The higher the number, the thinner the metal and the less expensive the casket (not to mention, easier for the pallbearers to carry). Funeral directors will frequently attempt to steer consumers away from the 20-gauge caskets—suggesting they are too thin and comparing them to an easily dented automobile fender made of similar gauge—and try, instead, to sell them the heavier, more expensive caskets.

Steel caskets are welded and the finish burnished and often spray painted. The linings, hardware, mattress, and other add-ons selected will, as with all caskets, have a direct bearing on the final price.

Frequently in lesser quality metal caskets, the bottom is not of the same material as the rest of the construction, and is merely spot welded to stay in place just long enough to be used once. While I'm told this is no longer the case, the spot-welded bottom was sometimes on caskets that were sold as sealed caskets. Who would know for certain? I don't recall any customers ever getting on their hands and knees and crawling under the casket to examine its underbelly construction.

Bronze and Copper—The finest caskets constructed of these materials are not welded; rather they are cast from molds (bronze and copper caskets comprise only about 3% of all caskets sold). Funeral directors are fond of referring to the bronze and copper (and sometimes even stainless steel) as "semiprecious metals"—a term I would find amusing were it not for the fact that it is a thinly veiled attempt to enhance the value of these caskets in the eyes (and pocketbooks) of the consumers. With these, as with all caskets, the "accessories" govern the final price.

Plastic, Aluminum, and Fiberglass Caskets— Caskets made of these materials are available, but not very popular (their combined sales are less than 1% of all casket sales). Of these, probably the plastic caskets have the longest life expectancy (wood rots and disintegrates, metal rusts and falls apart, plastic—as with the ubiquitous styrofoam cup—appears to last indefinitely).

Frequently, plastic caskets are used as liners inside more traditional caskets. Some funeral homes place a plastic liner casket inside a rental casket. When it comes time for interment, it is the plastic casket that goes into the ground. For sealing out intrusive elements, a hermetically sealed plastic casket undoubtedly ranks at the top. There is little aesthetic value to one of these, however, and the cost and accompanying profit are quite low; therefore, many funeral directors refuse to handle them. Just for the record, my own father is buried in a plastic casket.

Cardboard/Fiberboard Caskets—These are the least expensive of all caskets. Cardboard caskets are most commonly used for shipping remains across the country. Fiberboard caskets, those made of pressed wood fibers, are sometimes lined with cloth to dress them up a bit. Both are often used in cremations.

Specialty Caskets—Some casket manufacturers produce "specialty caskets" to appeal to perhaps the more irreverent and free-spirited of consumers. There are caskets designed to resemble automobiles, golf carts, boats, etc. A San Francisco company offers a line of unusual caskets including brightly colored ones, some in wild animal prints, others that are biodegradable, and another fashioned to look like an ancient sarcophagus.

A close friend in Columbus, Ohio, recently had to escort his just-widowed sister to select a casket. There, among the bronze and wood creations, was a scarlet and gray casket adorned with a sculpted cluster of buckeyes. For those of you familiar with the almost rabid allegiance of the area's fans to Ohio State University's football team (known, affectionately, as the Buckeyes and whose school colors are scarlet and gray), this casket probably doesn't come as a surprise. The deceased was one of those ardent fans. My friend and his sister selected another, more sedate casket—but, he admitted, they did waver just a bit!

It Pays to Shop Around

The Interfaith Funeral Information Committee (IFIC), a consumer-oriented non-profit agency founded in 1982, publishes an annual report on wholesale versus retail prices of funeral goods. In its report on 1995 prices, the

IFIC found the best deal was a 16-gauge bronze casket wholesaling for $6,550. The lowest retail price found by the IFIC was $6,750, while most other funeral homes were selling the same casket in the $16,375 to $19,650 range. The "prize" was taken, however, by the funeral home found by the IFIC to be selling that very same casket for $21,615—a *mere* profit of $15,065 (i.e., 330%).

Here are some of the IFIC's other 1995 findings:

• The *Autumn Oak* casket, manufactured by Batesville Casket Company (owned by Hillenbrand Industries which, by the way, also manufactures hospital furniture and American Tourister luggage), constructed of solid oak, wholesaled in mid-1995 for approximately $880 and retailed most commonly between $2,200 and $3,080, but was found to be selling for as high as $4,840.

• The *Franklin Silver* model, also manufactured by Batesville, a 20-gauge steel casket with a silver finish that wholesaled in mid-1995 for approximately $610 and retailed most commonly between $1,500 and $2,100, but on occasion as high as $3,965. By comparison, the company's *Primrose*, a pink steel model in 18-gauge steel, wholesaled for about $790, yet retailed between $1,975 and $2,765 and ran as high as $5,135. The firm's *India Star* silver model in 16-gauge steel wholesaled for $1,220 and was most commonly sold to the public for $3,050 and $3,660, but as high as $4,880.

• The *Crystal Blue* model by Batesville, manufactured in 18-gauge copper, wholesaled in mid-1995 for approximately $1,510; it retailed most commonly between

$3,775 and $4,530 but for as much as $6,040. A 16-gauge casket by the same company wholesaled and retailed for about $100 to $300 more.

Consumers Digest (September/October 1995) surveyed the wholesale and retail price sheets it obtained from major casket manufacturers. While the survey used the highest retail price found in each casket category, *Consumers Digest* pointed out that customers could purchase all of these products for less than half of the prices shown below:

Type	Retail	Wholesale	Profit
Cloth-covered	$500	$167	199%
Pine (solid)	$1,897	$749	153%
Oak (solid)	$2,600	$801	224%
Steel (16-gauge)	$2,255	$1,074	109%
Poplar (solid)	$3,050	$386	690%
Cherry (solid)	$3,550	$1,284	176%
Steel (stainless)	$4,050	$989	309%
Mahogany (solid)	$8,500	$1,810	369%
Bronze (48-ounce)	$31,000	$3,725	732%
Copper (solid)	$33,000	$1,625	1930%

The funeral homes owned by the conglomerates (more about them later) have an additional large-volume discount purchasing advantage. *Consumers Digest* pointed out that the conglomerate-owned businesses and other large-volume funeral homes can usually purchase these caskets for 25% less than the wholesale prices shown in this section.

Discounted caskets are becoming available. In Port St. Lucie, Florida, for example, a discount store selling caskets, vaults, and urns, offers a 32-ounce bronze casket for $2,900 that would probably cost the consumer $4,000 to $5,000 through a funeral director. When the store first opened, funeral homes countered the competition by tacking on a service charge (sometimes as high as $2,000) for caskets purchased elsewhere—a practice since made illegal by the FTC.

Sealer vs. Non-Sealer Caskets

Never underestimate the limits of ingenuity when fueled by greed. You would assume that, once you've made your selection from the incredibly wide array of caskets, you were done. Wrong. You must now choose between a "sealed" casket (also sometimes referred to as "gasketed" or "protective") and a "non-sealed" casket. Sealed with what? Sealed against what? And, pray tell, regardless of how good the warranty is, who's going to check to see if it leaked?

The majority of metal caskets (wooden caskets, because of the porous nature of wood, cannot be sealed) manufactured today are equipped with a neoprene gasket. After the lid of the casket is closed, the funeral director then turns internal screw mechanisms in the casket tightening the lid into a neoprene gasket. While federal regulations have greatly restricted the industry's

ability to claim that such devices protect the deceased—
sealing out water, insects, and vermin forever—the
implication is still quite strong in just the words: *protective
sealer*.

The truth is, our contemporary funeral practices (i.e.,
embalming, sealed caskets, and vaults) only delay the
inevitable and quite natural dust to dust, ashes to ashes
progression of human decomposition. These forces of
nature can be delayed for a time, but they cannot be
stopped.

Still, if such protection, even if only temporary, is
sufficient to persuade the consumer that the extra expense
is justified—there is another possible result. If the seal
does prove to be airtight (all seals, regardless of their
composition, will eventually disintegrate) while the body
completes its decomposition, the gases released by the
anaerobic bacteria—which actually thrive and multiply
faster in an airless environment—will have nowhere to
go. The abdominal cavity may bloat and even erupt, not
exactly the picture of eternal peace and protection
envisioned by the purchasing survivors. The gas pressure
can even be sufficient enough in some cases to explode
the seal around the lid of the coffin.

EERIE...BUT TRUE

Lest you think this is an apocryphal tale passed around at industry conventions, let me assure you it is not—this actually happened. Several weeks after a body was placed in a sealed casket and put into the mausoleum, the body exploded with such force that it destroyed the casket and blew the marble front off the crypt. A mortician was called in to clean up the pieces of the body and place them in a new casket, after which the crypt was repaired. Obviously, the family was never notified.

If mausoleum immurement is your choice, I strongly recommend against purchasing a sealing casket. If you have no option other than to purchase a sealing casket, then I urge you not to use the seal. For your information, coffins that are placed in mausoleums or above-ground crypts are routinely unsealed after the family leaves, just to relieve the inevitable buildup of gases within the casket and to prevent messy explosions. The families are none the wiser.

Bruce Armstrong, of the Armstrong Funeral Home in Canada, is among the growing number of death merchants maintaining World Wide Web sites on the Internet. Mr. Armstrong offers on-line this revealing scenario about discussing caskets and vaults with a friend named Hannie: "I explained to him that of all the caskets he saw in the room, there were basically only two types of caskets. Protective and non-protective caskets.

"Protective caskets…have a one-piece rubber gasket that runs around the entire lip of the casket. The head and foot panels have little pins that protrude and there is a steel wedge inside the lip of the casket. When the casket is closed, the pins go into the lip of the casket through openings in the gasket. We put a key (it's like a crank) into an opening at the foot end of the casket and turn it. This forces the steel wedge through the pins and causes the casket to seal at the rubber gasket.

"I showed Hannie a mirror under one of the caskets. He could see that there was a magnesium bar that is under the casket. I explained that when the casket starts to rust, electricity is generated. The electricity causes the magnesium to scab over the rust and the rust stops. It helps the casket last longer. The copper and bronze caskets don't have a magnesium bar because they will never rust.

"I began to show him the rust inhibitor which was applied to the inside of the casket and he said, 'Wait a minute, wait a minute! Who cares whether or not the casket rusts? Who cares about this protection thing? After all, the person is dead! Isn't this all a little extravagant?'

"I explained to Hannie that he wasn't realizing what the real product was that we were offering. He said, 'OK…what is the product?' I told him it was peace of mind. If a person felt more comfortable knowing that the body of the dead person was protected from the elements like water, gophers and so on, that option was available to them."

Mr. Armstrong ends his article with these telling words: "Having choices is what it's all about. After all, these people have to live the rest of their lives with the decisions that they make in an hour or two."

In some mortuaries, funeral directors are on a commission or some other performance-based bonus system that leads them to stress the importance of "protection" and to push for the sale of sealing caskets. Indeed, they are trained to try and sell a sealer casket and a sealer vault to each and every customer in order to "protect the loved one from the elements." This way, the industry makes certain prices—and profits—remain high.

Rent-a-Casket

If you're going to have a cremation but choose to precede it with a viewing, a casket will be necessary. But do you have to buy one for such a limited usage? No, rental caskets are generally available. Of course, the funeral director will try to steer you toward the purchase of a wood casket that can be incinerated along with the remains.

The industry is phasing out the rental business because it claims it generated insufficient profit. In the *Funeral Service Insider* newsletter (October 9, 1995), Bill Rice, of Sparkman-Hillcrest Funeral Home in Dallas, Texas, who stopped offering rentals in 1994, is quoted as saying, "We weren't doing well with rentals." He added that the growing number of attractive cremation caskets (the kind you burn up!) presents families with more choices.

The article compared the average $1,298 to $3,000 retail price of Rices's cremation caskets with the economics of his previous rentals. He revealed the wholesale cost of a rental casket was covered by the time it had been rented just two or three times. Although he offered that the casket would be rented eight or ten times (the casket's cloth-covered cardboard inserts were replaced after each use for a cost of $125), he must have concluded that a 700% profit paled in comparison to what he could make by selling the family a wooden one to be torched after just a few hours of viewing.

The article quoted others on the subject. Charles Monte of Chapel of the Hills Funeral Home in San Anselmo, California (the funeral home, according to the article, that handled the final arrangements for Jerry Garcia of Grateful Dead band fame), was quoted as saying rental caskets don't serve the family well. "There are no rentals or cloth in our line-up. If a family pays for (their loved one's) casket, it's only right, they own it," he explained. John McQueen of Anderson-McQueen Funeral in St. Petersburg, Florida (the firm that handled Mickey Mantle's funeral, according to the newsletter), said he stopped offering rental caskets since he made more money selling a cremation casket for $225 to $995 than renting one for $550, citing the cost of maintaining a rental as another reason.

Other funeral directors, though, said they found their cremation customers still preferred to rent, rather than buy, caskets. Dwight Hooper of Hooper Funeral Home in Inverness, Florida, solved the resulting cash crunch problem by simply raising the price of the rentals! There's always a way for those with a will.

Another article, headlined "Higher-end sales strategy wins points—so far," appeared in the *Funeral Service Insider* newsletter about a year later (January 15, 1996). It heralded the success of moving families toward purchasing, rather than renting, caskets. Following up, again with Mr. McQueen, the article said his firm had remodeled its cremation showroom and upgraded (i.e., raised prices on) the selection of caskets. The most expensive casket his firm stocked previously was listed at $995, but by utilizing the new approach, Mr. McQueen found that some customers were purchasing caskets costing as much as $2,600. "We take all families through our cremation showroom now," said Mr. McQueen.

Whose Vault Is it Then?

You've chosen burial and you've selected the appropriate casket, but you're still not done paying to have the body placed in the ground. A long way from it! If you've been to a graveside service, you're probably aware that the casket isn't placed directly in the soil. No. They've found another way to part you from more of your money. Though not required by law, vaults (or at least grave liners) are required by nearly every cemetery in the nation.

A grave liner, sometimes referred to as a "rough box," is a four-sided reinforced concrete box with no bottom and a loose-fitting lid. A vault, on the other hand, is a completely enclosed box and considerably more substantial. Both are lowered into the grave before the burial ceremony.

There are many styles of vaults, including unfinished concrete on which the concrete lid merely rests; concrete reinforced with steel; concrete coated with an asphalt mix with a grooved box and a flanged lid that fits into the groove; concrete with a metal, fiberglass, or plastic liner; and, more recently, plastic (or polypropylene) and fiberglass vaults.

Vaults can also be made of steel (either galvanized or nongalvanized and of 10-gauge or 12-gauge thickness). Steel vaults are the most expensive, carry the highest profit margin, and thus are the ones pushed hardest by the sales person.

Just what is a vault's purpose? As the consumer, you are told the vault offers additional—here comes that word again—protection! Yes, indeed. More protection from the insidious forces of nature: water, bugs, and those pesky gophers. For an additional cost, some vaults can be purchased with sealers.

This from an advertisement aimed at funeral directors for the Eagle Corinthian Burial Vault manufactured by Eagle Burial Vaults of Detroit, Michigan: "The quality and elegance usually reserved for higher priced vaults. Inspired by the strength and elegance that is classic Greek architecture, the Eagle Corinthian combines over sixty-five years of master craftsmanship with state-of-the-art technology. And like the great ancient columns, the Eagle Corinthian has been designed to offer the protection and durability that will stand the test of time... Consider the Corinthian, uniquely affordable, yet offering the peace of mind that is truly priceless."

Here we go again. Ad copywriters at their very best; creating attractive illusions that do not exist, yet staying within the boundaries of the law regarding deceptive advertising.

Before you consider making a sizable investment in a vault, please remember these three things: (1) the customer rarely ever sees the actual vault (it is normally selected from a catalog and it is already in the ground by the time the graveside ceremony takes place); (2) when the graves are closed, vaults are frequently damaged and even broken; and (3) just exactly how much craftsmanship and technology can there be in creating a vault?

And this from an advertisement for another vault manufacturer, Doric of Marshall, Illinois: "As your families deal with their grief, they shouldn't have to endure the added stress of choosing which burial vault is the strongest. That's why Doric vaults are built with strong protection for casketed remains... Doric vaults are modestly priced for value. And they have the lasting beauty of elegant hand-finishing as well as durability." Beauty? Hand-finishing?? These are simply concrete or metal boxes that are being planted in the ground and covered with dirt, ladies and gentlemen!

Perhaps my favorite, though, is the lyrical copywriting license taken in preparing the advertisement (as with the previous two, an advertisement speaking to funeral directors) for a new vault design by Wilbert, Inc., of Forest Park, Illinois: "Men call it cologne...Women call it perfume. Men say clothes...Women say fashion. Men buy mugs...Women buy stemware. Others call it a vault. We call it the Cameo Rose®. For decades Wilbert ® has been the leader in concrete burial vaults. Appealing as much to women as to men. But with the introduction of our new Cameo Rose, Wilbert maintains a universal design and enhances it with a distinctive feminine flair. A whisper of pink roses on a field of white and crowned with a personalized nameplate. Call it what you will, we call it the Cameo Rose." (Wow, that was exciting reading, wasn't it?)

No vault is impervious to eventual disintegration, and there is very little chance of placing anything underground and having it remain waterproof. I have personally witnessed as many as forty disinterments from vaults (even those made by the leading manufacturers) that were guaranteed waterproof from which water had to be drained before they could be moved. Often, they were full of water.

It's frequently necessary, when disinterring one of these vaults, to knock drainage holes in the bottom before it can be moved. Only then can the vault—still with the hole in the bottom—and casket be reinterred in another location. Occasionally a vault would actually prove to be too waterproof for a while. If there was excessive ground water, the vault would tend to float to the surface of the grave along with its contents. The solution, again, was very simple. Bring the vault up, knock some holes in the bottom, let the water fill it up, and sink it.

EERIE...BUT TRUE

The industry is filled with unique and eerie stories. One cemetery had a large sinkhole on the property. The sinkhole was 30 to 40 feet deep by the time it stopped growing. Apparently, the sinkhole drained into an underground cavern. Anyway, the hole encompassed a grave and the casket buried there was swallowed up by the hole and never seen again. There probably wasn't anything the cemetery operator could have done to prevent it.

They simply filled the hole back up, resodded, went about their business, and never informed the family.

So back to the justification for grave liners and vaults. Their original purpose was to discourage grave robbers. Grave robbing was a lucrative, if not attractive, profession for centuries. Long before there were legal means by which medical schools could obtain cadavers for anatomical dissection, the bodies were supplied by grave robbers—a practice which continued in the United States well into the 1900s. Grave liners and vaults were designed to make the grave robbers' work more difficult. Their success was directly tied to their ability to work quickly and quietly under cover of darkness. Nothing like a several-hundred-pound concrete lid to convince them they'd be better off moving to another grave site.

By the late 1920s, the supply of bodies to the medical schools increased and the need for grave robbers diminished. What to do with the grave liner and vault industries? Good old American ingenuity once again to the rescue.

To the delight of the products' manufacturers, the cemetery owners began requiring the installation of grave liners or vaults—heavy structures, often in excess of 2,000 pounds—in order, they said, to prevent the ground above the grave from caving in once the casket (that same casket supposedly "protecting" loved ones remains for an eternity if not longer) disintegrated. That's right. The sole purpose of grave liners and vaults is to prevent the ground above the grave from developing a small indentation when the casket collapses. This begs two fairly obvious questions:

(1) If caskets are being sold to protect the remains for the ages, why would there be a need for a grave liner or vault? Most caskets, certainly the ones constructed of steel or other metals, will last years before collapsing. In

fact, the landscaping "problem" may not even occur for generations to come. But let's get real here—

(2) Just exactly how much work does it take to fill in a slight depression in the soil and reseed it? I've done it several times in my own yard and I've not found the task terribly onerous, labor- or time-intensive, or expensive.

No. It is purely and simply another method to increase the sales and improve the profit margins. Depending upon the material, the quality of construction, and (as with caskets) any added extras, consumers can expect to pay from $200 to $400 for a grave liner, and from $300 to $10,000 for a vault. Spend it if you wish. But do so knowing full well that your investment is designed primarily to profit the seller and, secondarily, to assist the cemetery owners in their long-term lawn maintenance program. And please know that, over time, it will do precious little to protect the remains of the deceased.

Where you purchase a vault can make a considerable price difference. Cemeteries and funeral homes have had a long ongoing battle over the sale of vaults, each side lobbying for restrictions on the other. The profit motive is so strong that some have succeeded in having laws enacted that permit only funeral directors to sell vaults. I've had colleagues tell me that only funeral directors were qualified to sell vaults. Just exactly what type of qualification is required to sell a concrete box?

UNDERGROUND "CRYPTOMINIUMS"

Where states have barred cemeteries from selling vaults, the operators (not to be denied the opportunity to make a buck) have come up with a solution. They sell what are called "lawn crypts"—groups of multiple vaults pre-installed by the cemetery. They begin by excavating the ground to accommodate the vaults; as few as two and up to as many as several hundred may be constructed at one time. Drainage tile is installed, followed by a layer of gravel, and then the vaults are placed in the ground. The dirt is replaced, to be removed later as needed for burials. Lawn crypts are sold as being as dry as a mausoleum but at a much lower cost. In fact, however, the drains frequently clog and water must be pumped out of the vaults before the burial service.

Beyond this legislative horizon, there are also some questionable corporate restrictions. One of the major United States concrete vault manufacturers has an agreement with the funeral industry that its franchisees will sell the company's vaults *only* to funeral homes and *not* to cemeteries. The net effect of all these activities is to keep the price of vaults artificially high and to minimize competition. Consumers, for the most part, are completely unaware of the price manipulation and availability restrictions.

Vaults sold by cemeteries tend to be less expensive than those sold by funeral homes. Vaults sold by third-party vendors—where permitted by law—are generally the least expensive of all. Regardless of where they are purchased, all vaults do the same thing—they manage to keep the ground above the grave from sinking in, and they do not keep out water, nor do they prevent the natural decomposition of the body.

Monuments

Monuments, typically defined as above-ground memorials to the deceased, come in all shapes and sizes. They may be quite small—perhaps only four inches square—made of granite, marble, or bronze, installed flat on the ground, and cost as little as $200 or $300. Or they can be as large as 30 inches wide by 72 inches long (this size is referred to as a "ledger"), flat, and designed to cover the entire grave. A bronze ledger will cost the consumer approximately $6,000. Or monuments can be quite large, intricately carved sculptures costing many times that amount (the most expensive monument of which I'm personally aware cost the family $200,000).

The most economical place to purchase a monument is from a monument dealer or the funeral home, not the cemetery. Monument dealers and funeral homes, of course, need to make a profit. However, they do not pay the salespeople the inordinately high commissions that cemeteries seem to think they must in order to attract folks to that type of work. The savings by the monument dealers and funeral homes are usually reflected in lower prices to consumers. There are relatively few monument suppliers, and everyone—cemeteries, funeral homes, and monument dealers—must purchase from the same sources.

Cemeteries normally pay commissions that range from about 15% to 40%. They cannot compete, therefore, with the monument dealer or the funeral director who routinely will mark up the wholesale cost by only 15% to 25%. The cemeteries must rely on the consumer's lack of product knowledge and product availability, and employ high-pressure (usually in the customer's home) sales tactics to get the consumer to purchase from them.

Having been personally involved on both sides of this issue, I found it to be a continuing ethical debate. For example, a cemetery might sell a customer a monument for $1,500 and realize a $200 profit. On the other hand, the customer could go into a funeral home across the street and purchase the same monument for $900, and there will still be the same $200 profit.

The only answer I can give is that it is so difficult for cemeteries to hire, train, and retain qualified salespeople that they need to afford them every opportunity to make as much money as possible. So the prices of monuments sold by a cemetery need to be higher in order to pay the salesperson.

If you have already purchased a monument through a pre-need contract sold to you by a cemetery, I encourage you to check your contract and your state laws. In many instances, you can cancel this portion of the contract and be entitled to your money back (often with accrued interest). Do this and then do some comparison shopping at various monument dealers and funeral homes. Then repurchase the very same or equivalent memorial from one of them and I predict you can pocket several hundred dollars' worth of savings.

The Funeral Convenience Mart

As a consumer, you will find the funeral director able, and more than just a little ready and willing, to sell you a number of other conveniences in your time of need. If you are purchasing these during a time of grief and pressure, you will more likely be willing to pay the price of convenience. A convenience store sells the same bread and milk that a giant supermarket does, but the convenience store will do so at a cost of 25% to 50% more. I am going to run through some of the other "conveniences" that you may be offered by the funeral director. I only ask that you consider whether or not the additional price is worth it. Everything here you can purchase elsewhere by yourself for considerably less money.

Burial Clothing—Funeral directors will sell you clothing in which to bury your deceased. Professionally manufactured burial clothing is routinely of lower quality (it doesn't have to survive any washings or dry cleanings!) and often is made open in the back in order to facilitate placing it on the body. Most people, however, are buried in their own clothes and funeral directors will accommodate your wishes. Jeans, T-shirts, sneakers, suits, dresses, tuxedos, clown suits—whatever the family selects, the funeral director is bound to oblige. If a family feels the need for new clothing, they are better off—both from a fashion and budget sense—purchasing the clothes in a department store.

Flowers—In an attempt to capture yet another corner of the funeral market, some funeral homes maintain their own floral shops, or at least a very close and mutually beneficial liaison with a local florist. Suffice it to say that quality and price are most generally found elsewhere within the florist industry. As with all things we're discussing—whatever your choice, make it wisely and know you will save money if you shop elsewhere on your own.

Stationery—Granted, if you are purchasing funeral services on an at-need basis, you probably don't want to go shopping around for everything. Don't worry, the funeral director will be at your service, offering such marked-up items as guest registers, announcement cards, prayer cards, thank you cards, and acknowledgment notes. Could you purchase these yourself at a stationery store for less? Yes. Is the added convenience of *not* having to go the stationery store worth the added charges? Perhaps. Again, my purpose is only to inform you of your choices.

Vehicles—I'd imagine you'd like a hearse to pick up the body, deliver it to the funeral home, and then later to the cemetery? Me, too. Picking up a body without the right transportation equipment is difficult and awkward, and driving around town with it in the back seat is a little unseemly. By the time it's ready to go to the cemetery, the body's been "casketed" and is quite bulky and heavy. So a hearse is a good idea there, too.

But what about the other vehicles the funeral director may attempt to persuade you are necessary? Unless you're careful, you will receive—and pay for—a car to lead the procession to the cemetery, a limousine for the clergy and pallbearers, limousine(s) for you and your family, and a car to transport the flowers. You've agreed you need a hearse, but what are you other choices? Pallbearers, clergy, and family can certainly ride in personal cars; that's how they got to the funeral home isn't it? You can opt not to have the flowers at the graveside service, but you will probably still be charged for the removal and disposal of the flowers unless you make other arrangements.

Pallbearers—It is a solemn obligation but an honor to be asked to bear the casket of a departed friend or family member. Whenever possible, recruit your own. The funeral director, however, is able to furnish professional pallbearers if your personal situation warrants. While you're not likely to see a separate charge for the pallbearers listed on your funeral invoice, you should know the cost is being spread over the cost of other items you've purchased.

Recordings—Only in America! A growing trend among funeral directors is to offer the taping (video and/or audio) of the service. The premise behind this rather bizarre new marketing twist is to be able to share the event with family members unable to attend the service. If the idea appeals to you, I suggest having a trusted friend of the family do it for you at no cost.

Obituaries—There are two types of notices ("free obituaries" and "paid death notices") that appear in newspapers. Most metropolitan newspapers will, at no cost, print the obituaries of noteworthy (as so deemed by the newspaper) individuals. Indeed, newspapers write obituaries, often years in advance of a notable person's death, and update it as events warrant. These are known as "canned obits"—not something most people would regard as worthy notice of their status! Paid death notices, on the other hand, are furnished to the newspaper by the funeral home (in fact, to prevent practical jokes, most newspapers will accept death notices only from funeral homes). The longer the notice, the higher the cost. The funeral director can only pass on the cost to the consumer and not mark it up. I believe funeral homes should place these at no cost whatsoever to the consumer as they are, in fact, advertisements for the funeral home.

Death Certificate and Burial Permit—The funeral director is probably the best person to handle these necessary and unavoidable bureaucratic functions. The cost is minimal.

Cash Disbursements—In order to facilitate the planning and execution of the funeral service, the funeral director will need to make out-of-pocket expenditures for newspaper notices, flowers, clergy honoraria, gratuities, etc. Federal regulations prohibit the funeral director from profiting from these expenses without disclosing that fact to the consumer. Regardless, the consumer needs to maintain authority over such discretionary items.

Facilities and Professional Staff—There will be charges, of course, for the use of the funeral home, its furnishings, and its employees. Here is where much of the overhead of the funeral home is covered: visitation room, chapel, flower stands, lighting, kneeling benches, religious icons, the embalming/dressing/hair dressing of the deceased, staff to assist on visitations, staff and drivers to assist during the funeral and burial, etc. The most obvious way to save costs in this category would be to have the funeral service elsewhere (e.g., church or synagogue) and pay only for the costs of preparing and transporting the body.

Cemetery Charges—We've only been talking about the funeral director's charges so far. There are a number of additional expenses involved at the cemetery, such as burial plots, opening and closing the grave, memorials, mausoleums, perpetual care, and more. We will examine these in more detail later (see Chapter Five, *Graveyards to Memorial Gardens*).

EERIE...BUT TRUE

If I haven't convinced you to become a funeral director yet, read about these perks that could be yours. The Dead Ringer Putter Co., Inc., of Clifton Heights, Pennsylvania, offers casket-shaped cuff links, tie bars, and pendants (available in your choice of sterling silver or 14kt gold), ranging in price from $75 to $600. No well-dressed mortician would be caught dead with out 'em!

3

Death Merchants

How They Sell
What You May Not Want to Buy

"Funeral, n. A pageant whereby we attest our respect for the dead by enriching the undertaker, and strengthen our grief by an expenditure that deepens our groans and doubles our tears."
Ambrose Bierce, *The Devil's Dictionary* (1881-1911)

Indeed, the death merchants are enriched. But how do they do it? How are consumers, even in times of grief and panic, persuaded to part with so much money? It is not through chance, my friend. These are professionals at the art of selling and they work diligently and continuously to hone their craft.

The sales techniques utilized by the funeral directors differ in some ways from those used by the cemetery owners. We will examine them separately, but together they should empower you to make wiser, more studied, and sounder economic decisions.

On the Funeral Director's Turf

A subject of later discussion will be purchasing the funeral and disposition of the body on a pre-need basis (see Chapter Nine: *The Ins and Outs of Prearranging*). Even then, you will be subjected to the same skilled sales presentations, aided only by the fact you are not under any self-imposed pressure to make an immediate decision. The person making the same decisions on an at-need basis is considerably more vulnerable to being pressured into ill-advised purchases.

Consider for a moment something as supposedly innocuous as the funeral director's office. In the past, you've probably purchased a car or perhaps a house. It is highly unlikely that the car salesperson's cubicle or the realtor's office was ever constructed and decorated with so much forethought given to creating the right ambiance for closing a sale. At Slick Jack's Car Emporium, was there a picture of Jesus hanging on the wall above the salesperson's head? Was there a crucifix mounted next to the picture? Were there other religious symbols on the desk? Most probably not. Subtle, but not unpremeditated, nuances meant to persuade you that you are in a sacred place, not the sales office of a successful business. The atmosphere is crafted to be quasi-holy, an atmosphere in which you would experience pangs of guilt were you to question the decisions you were making or the prices you would have to pay for those decisions.

When you are on their turf, you are in the presence of selling elevated to scientific and artistic levels. The funeral and allied industries have studied and restudied the various ways in which to increase sales. Unless you are exceptionally well-prepared (and I hope this book will assist you toward that end) and unless you are emotionally strong and extraordinarily well-composed mentally and logically, you are at a distinct disadvantage. These professionals are the beneficiaries of decades of market research. They annually polish their sales skills at symposia and at regional and national trade shows. Assume that a death in your family occurs and no pre-arrangements have been made. You are under strict time constraints—not to mention, of course, the tremendous emotional stress—to make certain decisions. First, how to choose which funeral home?

Though funeral homes are required to give you price information over the phone, how inclined will you be to become a comparison shopper? Most people needing a funeral home operate on previous contact or referral. Perhaps you've attended a funeral at a particular establishment. Your family may have used a certain funeral home before (once a family has used a funeral home, the family historically continues to use that same funeral home, regardless of the cost). The funeral director may be known to you through a civic organization (funeral directors are known for their involvement in community affairs—perhaps it's due to an altruistic desire to help, but more often it is born out of a need for marketing). Barring those experiences, you may wish to turn to your clergy for advice because, if you can't trust the judgment and counsel of your clergy, there are probably few others you can trust, right?

HOOKED ON HIS PROFESSION

Because of funeral directors' typically high profiles within their communities (through their involvement in schools, civic and fraternal organizations, etc.), many believe them to be people of high integrity and trust. Similarly, most would assume that funeral directors must have a well-developed sense of self-esteem. That's not always the case.

Several years ago, a funeral director who worked for me shared this story. He had just come out of a long and bitter divorce. He was on the road, feeling lonely, and decided to engage the services of a prostitute. When the hooker showed up in his hotel room, she asked for some identification to convince her he was not an undercover police officer.

First, he showed her his driver's license, but she said that wasn't proof enough. He proceeded to sort through other types of identification he carried in his wallet and produced his funeral director's license. She took one look at the card and then flatly refused to have sex with him. He pleaded with her and even offered her more money, but to no avail. She turned and walked out of the room. Sometimes funeral directors don't get any respect!

In 1994, the Interfaith Funeral Information Committee released a study of the funeral industry that addressed this subject. According to the report, some members of the clergy may have relationships with funeral directors that involve what can only be described as bribery: gifts, gratuities, and inflated funeral service honoraria for making referrals to certain mortuaries. Also, it is far too common a practice for funeral directors to pay money to hospital and emergency personnel to send bodies to their funeral homes. The funeral industry is aware that once a body is inside their mortuary, there is at least a 95% chance the family will leave the body there for preparation and services. Therefore, the motive of greed frequently overwhelms common sense and ethical behavior.

MAKING THEM FEEL HEARSE

For decades, prior to the adoption of training and licensing requirements for paramedics, funeral homes routinely provided emergency transportation for the ill and injured. They had the staff and the vehicles to perform the job. The truth, of course, is that providing this service put them first in line to get the body in case of a death. Drivers must have felt a conflict of interest when they caught themselves hoping their passenger would die en route so they wouldn't have to make two trips!

The study detailed such examples as offering ministers and priests country club memberships, free vacations on mortuary aircraft, and tickets to major sporting events. These are the blatant examples. The less obvious, however, are still done with the identical purpose of increasing referrals: calendars, appointment books, charitable and in-kind contributions, etc. All are considered "advertising" by the funeral industry which understandably takes umbrage at the mere suggestion that such efforts are unethical.

In a July 1994 edition of the *Arizona Republic* newspaper, Jack Botimer, a 37-year veteran of the funeral business, manager of the Botimer Family Mortuary, and an outspoken critic of his own industry, was quoted as saying of such advertising, "It is a built-in expense for the industry. It is especially a problem here in Phoenix, where so many people have come from somewhere else. Back in their hometown, maybe everyone knew the mortician. Transplanted here," he said, "they depend on a clergyman to refer them to a mortuary." He added, "I know of no mortuary that will admit it, but they all try to bribe the clergy whenever then can. On the other hand, I've had clergymen demand a certain amount for a funeral—from as high as $100—and expect me to collect it from the family. I won't do it." He was also quoted as saying, "It has been my experience that the majority of the clergy are as naïve and poorly informed about the funeral industry as the average parishioner."

So what are you supposed to do? Your deceased loved one is lying in the bed upstairs or maybe at a nearby hospital. Time's running out. You make a choice, dial the phone, and arrange for the body to be taken to a mortuary. Now you must go yourself and make those infamous "final arrangements."

The best advice in this situation is don't go alone. Take someone with you to the funeral home, such as a friend, an adviser, perhaps your attorney or accountant, or even your pastor or priest, but certainly someone who is not caught up in the emotional crisis of the moment. Take someone upon whom you can rely for dispassionate counsel, even if that person is not knowledgeable of the funeral industry and the pricing of its goods and services.

Be advised, however, that the funeral director already knows more about you and your financial situation than you may want to realize. If your family has been served previously by the mortuary, then your family's spending preferences and credit standing are a matter of record.

NOT PSYCHIC...JUST NOSEY

Commonly, sales goals are simply based on the customer's first phone call to the funeral home. Just by giving your home address, the funeral director is aware of the real estate values in your neighborhood. This assumption becomes knowledge once the mortuary staff is present to remove the body, taking due note of your house, its furnishings, and even your automobiles. By the time you arrive at the funeral home, the funeral director is prepared to sell to the limit of what he perceives to be your financial capabilities.

The Trip to the Mortuary

Alone or not, there you are at the mortuary. What can you expect to see? What can you expect to hear? What decisions will you need to make?

After the funeral director's condolences and muted pleasantries designed to impart empathy and to put you at ease, you will be asked for certain vital information to assist in procuring the death certificate. You should be prepared to provide date of birth, social security number (which, by the way, will enable the funeral director to electronically check your credit standing), and other pertinent personal information. Also, you will be asked about insurance information which will put the final piece into the financial puzzle the funeral director has been assembling.

In my experience, even those in the lower socio-economic strata often have a $5,000 or $10,000 life insurance policy. Often it is the funeral directors' goal to have the consumer assign that insurance policy directly to the funeral home to guarantee payment. Of course, it is also their goal to try and sell enough goods and services to use up as much of the insurance benefit amount as possible. They do this by telling the family that this was the last demonstration of love they could give the deceased. They do this by stressing that this was surely what the deceased would have wanted, emphasizing that's why the deceased had the insurance in the first place. And, soon after the family leaves the office, the funeral director will call the insurance company and verify the policy, rather than finding out a month or two later there might be a problem.

Securing payment is sometimes difficult. I know from my own experience that we had to return grave markers to customers who refused to pay us for the installation. In other instances of non-payment for mausoleums, we moved bodies from the crypts and buried them in cheaper in-ground graves. If insurance monies are not available and there is doubt about the consumer's credit, funeral facilities will sometimes require full payment in cash in advance before they will inter the body.

During your meeting with the funeral director, you will be asked many questions about your family and about the deceased's personality, interests, career, religion, memberships in civic organizations, and hobbies. These are not designed merely to be friendly and understanding of your needs. Instead, they are designed to elicit information to enable the funeral director to guide you to greater and more expensive purchases.

Next, you will be asked to decide what type of services you desire. Visitations? Open or closed casket? Service at a church or synagogue or—preferably, as far as the funeral director is concerned—at the funeral home? Interment? And you will be offered the array of amenities we discussed earlier (e.g., limousines, flowers, stationery, etc.). Once these questions are answered, you will be provided with a written price list detailing all of the expenses you've authorized. Take your time and read it carefully, for it is a binding contract. Ask questions (easier said than done, I realize—but this is the time to remove any remaining doubt and to make any changes necessary to get the services you want and can afford).

If you are going to have the deceased embalmed, you should also bring with you to the funeral home clothing for burial, and any other items you wish the deceased to wear (e.g., jewelry, wig, and—yes—even false teeth!). Also, a recent photograph of the deceased is exceptionally helpful to the person doing the embalming and restoration—to aid in creating what funeral directors are fond of calling the "memory picture."

Fiery Cremation Sales Tactics

But, you tell the funeral director, you desire a direct cremation (or, for that matter, a direct burial)—no embalming, no visitations, no service. How might these wishes be countered? (For a more detailed discussion of the cremation process itself, please see Chapter Four: *The Question of Cremation.*) You should be aware that the funeral industry is working mightily to widen the profit margins associated with cremations.

Funeral directors long considered cremations to be an anathema to their business, a veritable threat to their livelihood. As the number of cremations increased, however, the industry learned to adapt and to promote additional services and goods to accompany cremations. For a number of years, crematories even got away with charging families a fee for releasing the cremains to them! The Federal Trade Commission abolished this practice, saying that by merely providing cremation services that the crematories did not acquire any rights to the ashes (now that's reassuring!).

Undaunted, the industry continues to move forward in its insatiable quest for greater profits. Direct from the *Funeral Service Insider (FSI)* (October 9, 1995) come some suggestions on how to boost cremation profits:

• Ask families what kind of a cremation they want, for most are unaware that cremation can involve more than simply sending the body to the crematorium. By initiating such a conversation and describing various alternatives, funeral directors may be able to sell a wider variety of goods and services.

• Ask the families if they had a chance to see their loved one before he or she died; then ask them if they'd like to see the person again before a direct cremation. This opens the door to selling them on the idea of embalming and other related items.

• Offer only metal rental caskets, since rental caskets are not a money-maker. Consumers generally find metal caskets unappealing and will often choose to purchase more expensive wood caskets rather than rent metal ones.

• Offer the family a wide range of options—from an inexpensive cremation tray to a much more costly oak casket to a wide selection of urns. Many funeral directors believe that if there are many choices, the family will frequently opt for more rather than less in the way of merchandise and services.

Some funeral directors have started giving a printed information sheet to clients who are considering cremation. This propaganda stresses how important the viewing of the deceased is to the grieving process. It helps families and friends, they say, to cope with the death.

At many funeral homes, cremation urns are on display so the customers can handle them and get a feel for them. Some funeral directors have even constructed altars, complete with lighted candles, to show how the urn would look during the service they are hoping the customer will buy. Also, many funeral directors place price tags on the bottom of the urns so the customers will focus on the "character and quality" and not on the price.

Perhaps the most telling advice for persuading people to spend more than they intended was contained in another issue of the *Funeral Service Insider* newsletter (September 25, 1995): "What's your best bet for personalizing cremation services—and steering families away from direct disposition? Guide your arrangement conference toward the subject of doing something for the young grandchildren or children of the deceased. 'That can really change the dynamics of a cremation arrangement,' says Ric Newton, co-owner of Newton-Bracewell-Chico (California) Funeral Home." Even if they're leaning toward little or no ceremony, "the parents become very receptive to anything dealing with children," he said. And that can lead to big upgrades from direct disposition—embalming, visitations, funeral and memorial services, and better urns and cremation containers, says Newton. The newsletter offered this "tip" to funeral directors: "Start by suggesting that children be allowed to draw 'goodbye pictures' for their deceased grandparent or parent. Then suggest showing the pictures on an easel during the service."

I rest (at least momentarily) my case. Let us return to the casket room—our next stop on your visit to the funeral home.

A Tisket, A Tasket—So *That's* How They Sell Caskets

Lest you think the display of caskets was the result of random, haphazard placement, please reconsider. Some casket manufacturers actually reserve the right to approve the showroom, and some require funeral homes to carry a minimum of 70% to 80% of that particular manufacturer's caskets as a prerequisite for being allowed to sell its line and to qualify for the manufacturer's discount. The funeral directors, and particularly the manufacturers, have worked long and hard, experimenting with casket layouts, testing them through consumer research, and refining the placement, pricing, and presentation of the caskets.

Different methods have been tested and tried over the years. In his book *Successful Funeral Management*, W.M. Krieger suggested discarding the idea of placing the caskets in a row from least to most expensive. Such an arrangement (he referred to it as the "stairstep" method) enabled the consumer to make price comparisons too easily. Instead, he recommended an approach which divided the arrangement of caskets into fourths, two of them above a certain median price and the other two below it, with the goal to sell a casket just above the median price. The consumer would first be shown a casket in one quadrant priced above the median and higher than the budget discussed. If the consumer said it was too expensive, the next casket shown would be in a second quadrant and considerably less expensive and also of lesser quality. The funeral director would be betting that the consumer would say the lesser casket was insufficient and would then lead him to the "rebound" casket located in a third quadrant and priced just below the price of the first casket shown. The "rebound" casket was the one initially targeted for sale by the funeral director, but the consumer was led to feel that he or she was in charge of the whole process. Complicated, but he was convinced it worked.

The "triangle" method is similar in that the consumer is unaware of the manipulation taking place. The room is laid out with caskets displayed in triangular groupings. Beginning at one point of the first triangle, the consumer is shown a casket selling, for example, for $1,975, but is told that it is in the $1,500 to $2,000 range. The next casket shown sells for $2,225, but our consumer is told that it is just $250 more. If no negative reaction is received after being shown either casket, the consumer would then be led to another triangle where the prices are proportionately higher and the cycle would begin again. If, however, the consumer balked at the higher of the two caskets in the first triangle, the funeral director would lead the way to the third casket, selling for $2,025 and be told that the savings would be $200.

Most standard methods for selling caskets are based on the premise that the average consumer is most likely to purchase in the middle of the casket price range. The consumer may not purchase the most expensive casket, but simply by having it present, the consumer is more apt to find the mid-priced casket more reasonable by comparison. Conversely, the consumer will not want to consider the least expensive caskets of obviously inferior quality. To capitalize on these assumptions, the funeral directors will show the most and least expensive caskets first.

The casket salesperson is an adaptable sort! If it is perceived that "protection" is important to the consumer, then that will be the focal point of the presentation and metal caskets will be shown. If, however, the consumer mentions something about the beauty of wood, then the sales pitch will smoothly shift gears to extol the virtues of wood and no more mention of "protection" will be made. The buyer, of course, will later hear the funeral director stress the qualities of the more expensive sealing vaults in order to "protect" the beautiful wood casket just selected.

Another common ploy is to show only the more expensive casket, even if you have a similar model available for a lower price. Funeral directors know that people tend to choose what's on display. Often, consumers will find a selection of caskets whose prices escalate in $100 to $200 increments. This, too, is by design, for funeral directors have learned that people are more easily led to the higher priced caskets if the price differentials are not considered too great.

There are many other sales devices that may be used. Frequently, the least expensive caskets on display are of an unattractive color. Perhaps the lining is not matched to the color of the casket, or the lesser caskets may have scratches or other obvious surface defects. They may be displayed on the lowest shelf to make them appear (at least subconsciously) as inferior. The whole purpose is to make it difficult to envision the loved one reposing in such an unbecoming structure and to gently but firmly lead the consumer up the casket price ladder!

Once the initial conference and the tour of the casket room is complete, the funeral director may attempt to separate you from any non-family adviser you might have brought along. The feeling of the funeral director, of course, is that you and your family will arrive at more extensive/expensive decisions if left alone to ponder the size of your final tribute. Don't let this happen. It is precisely at this point that you need objective input to help you continue to think clearly and make the wisest choices.

4

The Question of Cremation

How to Arrange a Cremation without Getting Burned

"As well a well-wrought urn becomes/ The greatest ashes, as half-acre tombs."
John Donne, "The Canonization," *Songs and Sonnets* (1633)

Humans have cremated their deceased throughout recorded history and even before. Civilizations from the ancient Australians, Babylonians, Greeks, and others have used the funeral pyre to literally invoke the "ashes to ashes" concept of death. In *I Samuel* (31:12-13) of the Bible you can read, "All the valiant men arose, and went all night, and took the body of Saul and the bodies of his sons from the wall of Beth-shan, and came to Jabesh, and burnt them there. And they took their bones, and buried them under a tree at Jabesh, and fasted seven days."

BONFIRE

The word "bonfire" is derived from the Middle English word "bonefyre" meaning, literally, a fire of bones. The word denoted the funeral pyre. Think about *that* the next time you're roasting marshmallows!

Cremation fell out of vogue in most modern civilizations by the 17th to 18th centuries. By the late 1800s, however, against a backdrop of public protest, cremation advocates—particularly in Europe—began to promote the burning of the dead. They cited concern for the public health and about the pollution of the environmental groundwater they feared was being caused by in-ground burials. The frontiersmen of the American West were also known to use cremation on occasion if the following verse by Robert Service (*The Cremation of Sam McGee*, 1907) is any indication:

> *The Northern Lights have seen queer sights*
> *But the queerest they ever did see*
> *Was that night on the marge of Lake Lebarge*
> *I cremated Sam McGee.*

By the turn of the century, cremation was becoming more accepted as an alternative to burial. The proponents offered many persuasive arguments: (1) land was too scarce in many areas to be given over for the burial of the dead; (2) cemeteries would be sources of pollution even decades after the final interment; (3) cremation replicates the exact same process that a buried body will undergo, just far more quickly and without the unpleasant images of slow decomposition; and (4) a cremation is far less expensive than a full funeral service and subsequent burial.

Another argument was proffered around that same time. It was suggested that cremation would prevent any possibility of being buried alive (many don't realize it, but the fictional tales of Edgar Allan Poe were very real fears to the people of that time). On the other hand, the cremation advocates made no mention, however, of the fear of possibly being burned alive! Also, proponents argued, cremation would eliminate the very real concern that the remains of loved ones would be violated by grave robbers—another very real concern of the time.

Kenneth V. Iserson, M.D., in his book *Death to Dust* (1994, Galen Press, Ltd.) cites an early American pro-cremation pamphlet as depicting the choice between burial and cremation as, "between incineration which disposes the body in one hour in a beautiful glow of heat, and earth burial which prolongs the process through fourteen to twenty years of loathsome decay."

Cremations on the Increase

Cremation is slowing gaining acceptability in the United States. As low as 6% in 1975 and 15% in 1985, cremations topped 20% of dispositions in 1994 for the first time in history. Industry forecasters predict that the figure will exceed 30% of dispositions by the year 2010.

CREMATION HEATING UP

The choice of cremation over burial in the United States varies widely according to the regions of the country. If you subscribe to the theory that the majority of our fads and fashions begin on the coasts and work their way to the center of the nation, then you will be led to believe that cremations will become the norm, rather than the exception, for the disposition of our dead in the future. As a percentage of cremations to deaths, here are the figures shown by geographic region and by year:

REGION	ACTUAL			PROJECTED		
	1992	1993	1994	1995	2000	2010
New England	20.68	21.83	23.81	25.27	32.80	46.13
Mid-Atlantic	15.18	15.74	16.46	17.12	20.37	26.59
East North Central	15.13	16.32	17.26	18.34	22.98	30.53
West North Central	12.18	12.36	13.35	14.30	18.34	25.38
South Atlantic	18.88	21.04	21.23	22.13	25.41	30.44
East South Central	3.62	3.88	4.65	4.82	6.46	9.10
West South Central	7.92	8.87	9.55	10.17	13.13	17.62
Mountain	35.53	36.83	35.63	37.94	42.29	48.10
Pacific	43.52	41.76	43.37	44.05	47.21	52.70
United States	**19.11**	**19.78**	**20.60**	**21.49**	**25.19**	**31.28**

Source: *Cremation Association of North America*

What Exactly Happens in a Cremation?

Although it is perfectly acceptable (not to mention, cheaper) to use nothing at all, most bodies that are cremated are either on, or in, something combustible. Heavy cardboard trays, cardboard or wood caskets, and even canvas body bags are most commonly utilized. Metal containers are not used as they would actually bake the body, rather than incinerate it. In busier crematories, a non-flammable tag with the deceased's name is placed with the body to guarantee accurate identification of the remains following cremation. Less busy crematory operators rely on their good judgment to remember just who it was they cremated.

The doors to the cremation oven, or "retort" as it is called in the industry, are opened and the body slid inside. The retort is then heated to approximately 1,000° to 1,500° Fahrenheit. While some retorts are manufactured to operate on liquid propane or electricity, most are fueled by natural gas.

From your days in high school biology and physiology, you may recall that most parts of the human body—muscle tissues, flesh, and organs—are composed primarily of water (70-80%), and the balance of bones composed primarily of calcium phosphate. The application of the intense heat of cremation first evaporates the water from the body. The flames then incinerate the muscles, flesh, and organs. Most of the bone structure will crumble, but will not be reduced to ashes, by cremation.

The actual incineration process takes an average of one to two hours, depending on the temperature inside the retort, the condition and size of the corpse (the bodies of obese individuals give off considerable black smoke and flames when incinerated and take longer to cremate than more slender folks), and on the type of container used. The Environmental Protection Agency has required crematories to install expensive but effective scrubbers to their smokestacks to prevent any of the smoke or residue from cremation to escape into the surrounding atmosphere.

Once the process is complete and the oven has cooled, an attendant uses (*note to pizza lovers*: please excuse the following analogy) a brush similar to those used to clean pizza ovens to remove the ashes and bone fragments, and sometimes a vacuum cleaner is used. We will, here forward, use the euphemism promoted by the funeral industry and refer to these ashes and bone fragments as "cremains." The cremains are then placed in a box or in an urn purchased by the family.

How much is left and what do the cremains look like? The average man, when cremated, yields approximately six to seven pounds of cremains and the average woman five to six pounds. The cremains are generally gray in color but can contain flecks of other colors created by jewelry, dental fillings, etc.

If the ashes are to be scattered, the cremains will most probably be passed through a pulverizing machine to grind the bones to a consistency similar to that of the rest of the ashes (some crematory operators routinely pulverize all cremains). What results has the granular consistency of sand and bears no resemblance at all to human remains.

In the pulverization process, it is inevitable that some small amount of residue from other cremains will be mixed with others and some of the cremains may be lost, but the amounts are likely to be minuscule. The possibility of having the cremains of loved one commingled with those of someone else is quite small. In the past, it was not unheard of for a crematory to incinerate more than one body at a time (always concerned about that darned profit margin, those little devils!), but substantial awards resulting from successful lawsuits makes such a risk by a crematory totally unacceptable unless authorized in writing by the persons requesting a multiple cremation.

Can you witness the cremation? Crematory policies vary, but the standard response is no. The reason, the operators say, is one of liability. The truth is, crematory operators would rather not have to deal with the emotionally distraught in front of the flaming retort, nor do they want to risk having people disseminate misinformation about the actual cremation process (always remember, the funeral and cemetery industries achieved, and they maintain, much of their clout through secrecy). They will attempt to dissuade you by suggesting the procedure is too technically complicated to comprehend and that you are most probably not psychologically prepared to handle it. But if this is your desire, call around until you can locate a crematory willing to oblige your wishes. Be prepared, however, to sign an insurance waiver designed to protect the crematory from later being charged with inflicting emotional distress.

You Got Those Cremains the Old-Fashioned Way... You *Urned* Them

If you've not already purchased an urn, or have chosen not to, the cremains will be given to you in a plastic container or a cardboard box. Perhaps you've decided to scatter the ashes at some place of personal significance, in which case an urn really isn't necessary. There are few laws that prohibit the scattering of ashes. Indeed, some cemeteries (bless their management's mercenary hearts) have established "scattering areas" on their properties where a family can strew the cremains—for a fee, of course. And there are services (for hire) that will scatter cremains from ships or aircraft over the site selected.

EERIE...BUT TRUE

One particular decedent had chosen cremation and left directions that his ashes were to be strewn over his favorite fairway at his country club. The survivors chose an appropriate morning and gathered at the golf course.

While a foursome of golfers waited patiently to tee off, the five family members took turns dipping their hands into the box, scooping out the cremains, and tossing them into the gentle spring breeze. I don't believe they were aware ahead of time that the box would contain nearly seven pounds of cremains—that's a lot! The airborne ashes drifted to the ground and made about a fifty-foot gray circle on the dew-covered fairway. But, determined and committed to their task, they continued.

A fresh wind picked up and began blowing the ashes back toward the family members. By the time they were finished, their hands and clothes were covered with the gentleman's ashes. They probably wanted to feel close to him by fulfilling his wishes through this solemn ritual, but not quite that close!

The selection of urns grows wider each year as more designs are added by manufacturers hoping to capitalize on the trend toward more cremations. Urns are available in copper, wood, steel, bronze, marble, ceramic, glass, and even plastic, and in secular and non-secular designs, classic styling, and modern. There are vertical urns and horizontal urns. The choices are seemingly endless. They come in a variety of sizes: adult, child, and infant. And, for those who don't believe in "till death do us part" there are combination urns, designed to hold separately, or commingled, the cremains of a couple.

Many cemeteries require urns be placed in a vault if the cremains are to be buried. Thought you were saving money by selecting a cremation, were you? One manufacturer advertises its cremains burial vaults, constructed of high-impact polystyrene, as providing "Embarrassment Protection" (I don't know what that is, and I'm not at all certain I *want* to know!).

Even though I was in the business for thirty years, I am still amazed at the ingenuity of the providers to the death business and the lengths to which they will go to create new products to increase sales. For example, a Wisconsin company offers jewelry—lockets in the shapes of hearts and crosses—in which to place tiny bits of cremains. They also sell, as an alternative, glass bell jars in which to suspend the lockets in the event you don't wish to have ol' Uncle Larry hanging around your neck.

Perhaps the award for the most creative new product, though, should go to the manufacturer in Illinois that is now offering hollow, blown-glass urns in "twelve designs with cremains visible, permanently embedded in glass." As only a small portion of the cremains are used in one urn, the maker suggests that now family members can each have their own urn! Now that's a way to increase sales—sell an urn to every member of the family!

How Much Should Cremation Cost?

Consumers Digest (September/October 1995) reported on its cremation-related survey of 12 major markets coast to coast in the United States. The most competitive prices, the magazine found, were offered by memorial societies and alternative providers, as opposed to funeral homes (no surprise there!). For a direct cremation (i.e., one with no embalming, viewing, service, or premium products) the average cost was approximately $490. The lowest price ($390) in the magazine's survey was found in both Chicago and Pittsburgh, and the highest ($690) was reported in both Boston and Baltimore.

Remember, however, these are *average* costs for a *direct* cremation. As I mentioned in the preceding chapter, funeral directors are trained to sell the cremation "extras" (e.g., embalming, viewing, etc.). A Grosse Point, Michigan, funeral director reports that the cremation bill at his establishment averages $3,600 when all the amenities he talks his clients into are tallied. Quite a contrast to the $390-$690 range shown above.

5

Graveyards to Memorial Gardens

The Ingenuity of Interment

*"Dust to dust, ashes to ashes, and the cremains to a memorial park.
All this is supposed to maintain the dignity of death."*
Joseph Wood Krutch, the title essay, 1,
If You Don't Mind My Saying So (1964)

So far we've primarily discussed funeral homes and crematoria, but cemeteries and memorial gardens are also very big businesses in the United States. Through a combined exploitation of the tax laws and manipulation of the consumer, operators of these establishments oversee a billion-dollar industry.

Bone up on Boneyard Definitions

Cemeteries—The word "cemetery" comes from the German words "koimeterion" (a sleeping place) and "koiman" (to put to sleep). These word origins fit in well with the industry's aversion to the word "death," preferring instead to allude to an eternal slumber. Cemeteries are, quite simply, a place to bury the remains of the dead. There are many types of cemeteries, including church graveyards, private cemeteries, public cemeteries, commercial cemeteries, and national cemeteries for veterans. Within them, grave markers range from the simple plaque on the ground to quite large and elaborate statuary. Burial sites range from a hole in the ground to large above-ground structures. Maintenance of the cemeteries ranges from the nonexistent to funded plans to ensure such care for perpetuity. Here are some brief descriptions of the different types of cemeteries:

Church cemeteries were among the first formal cemeteries in our country. Churches would put together a small cemetery for their parishioners, usually adjacent or quite close to the church itself. Over the years, many of these cemeteries have fallen into disrepair due to a number of factors: the church might have hard financial times and lacked the funds necessary to maintain the cemetery, the church might have gone out of existence altogether, or the church might have flourished and moved to a new location. Typically, churches are tax-exempt and their cemeteries are not covered by any of the state laws concerning perpetual care.

Private cemeteries, also known as family cemeteries, were as common as church cemeteries until well into the 20th century, particularly in rural areas. It was common for families to bury their deceased on a hillside or somewhere behind the house on the property they owned. Times have changed. Families are considerably more mobile than their ancestors, and the old family cemeteries are frequently neglected if not forgotten completely. My own grandparents are buried in such a family cemetery. For a long time, we used to get a group together every two or three years and go in and clean up the cemetery.

Now we simply pay someone else to do the maintenance. In most areas of the country, private cemeteries are still permitted, but the long-term outlook for care and maintenance of such grave sites is not encouraging.

Public cemeteries, also often referred to community cemeteries, have also been around for a long time. Founded with good intentions by city and village councils, these cemeteries often lack sufficient funding to operate efficiently and provide adequate maintenance. Exacerbating the problem is the fact that many of the older cemeteries are, as is the case with church-run cemeteries, exempt from state laws governing perpetual care. While the original intentions might be considered commendable, is it the role of government to tax all its citizens in order to provide burial spaces below going market rates? I realize it's my political and past professional bias, but I don't believe the role of government is to be in competition with free enterprise.

Memorial Gardens (also referred to as *Memorial Parks*)—Memorial gardens are cemeteries, but with the distinction that the grave markers are frequently uniform in size, flat, and set flush with the ground. The perception upon entering a memorial garden is one of a large, meticulously landscaped and manicured park. One of the purported purposes for such flat markers is to minimize the trimming of grass, thereby reducing the cost of labor in maintaining the cemetery. The invention of string grass trimmers and lawn mowers that can cut flush with upright structures hasn't changed the way memorial gardens are run, however.

Columbaria—A columbarium is a pretty word meaning a vault, a room, or sometimes just a wall with niches in which to place urns containing the cremains.

Columbaria can range from the quite simple, but tastefully dignified, to ornate structures of bronze and imported marble. Urns can be placed behind stained or etched glass in niches complete with subdued indirect lighting within rooms filled with soft, prerecorded music. The older custom of keeping a loved one's ashes at home (a great conversation starter, by the way) is persuasively discouraged as bordering on necrolatry (defined as an excessive reverence for the dead).

Cremation Gardens—These are separate areas of cemeteries set aside for the below-ground burial of urns. Typically, the cemeteries require the urns to be in a vault (as though the remains are going to further decompose and cause those large, unsightly depressions in the ground). And, again, there may be *scattering gardens*, areas of the cemetery reserved for families to strew the ashes of the deceased.

Mausoleums—Mausoleums are tombs sometimes of extraordinary splendor (the Taj Mahal, for example, is a mausoleum), often built for the prominent, the wealthy or, at the very least, the egocentric. While the word "crypt" historically meant a below-ground burial chamber, the cemetery industry now refers to the chambers within above-ground mausoleums as crypts.

The price for crypts depends upon location. Typically, crypts will be named in some manner. Commonly, the bottom crypt is called the "Prayer Level," the next up is the "Heart Level," then the "Eye Level," and the highest is called the "Heaven Level." The prices are higher for the Eye Level and Heart Level crypts than for the others, as you don't need to stoop or stretch to touch the door of the crypt as many like to do.

Many cemeteries offer a selection of "cryptic" possibilities: *community mausoleums* that hold large numbers of caskets, often in walls surrounding a chapel-like room with stained-glass windows; *family mausoleums* for the families who like to do absolutely everything together; and *private mausoleums* for those who prefer to be alone for truly extended periods of time! Some larger mausoleums are even decorated with furniture, paintings, and photographs and other mementos of the deceased. There are other choices as well: *end-to-end* (i.e., deep crypts into which two caskets are inserted one after the other), *side-by-side* (i.e., wider crypts into which two caskets are placed next to each other), and *couch* (i.e., crypts in which caskets are placed sidewise).

SARCOPHAGUS

The word "sarcophagus" is derived from the Greek word "sarkophagus"—a combination of two words: "sarkos" meaning flesh and "phagein" meaning to eat. At a loss to explain the decomposition of their deceased, ancient peoples decided it was caused by the stone coffins in which their dead were buried. They believed it was the stone coffin itself that was devouring the corpses.

National Cemeteries

The National Cemetery System (NCS) is currently comprised of 114 cemeteries located in 38 states and in Puerto Rico, and will operate on an annual budget of $76.2

million in fiscal year 1997. There are also Arlington National Cemetery (managed by the United States Army) and 24 overseas military cemeteries (run by the American Battle Monuments Commission). National cemeteries have been around for a long time, created by Congress and signed into law by President Abraham Lincoln. The original purpose was to provide proper burial for soldiers killed in the Civil War.

In the past 20 years, annual interments in national cemeteries have nearly doubled to over 70,000 per year and the rate of increase is projected to continue into the early part of the next century as our country's population of military veterans grows older. Many of these cemeteries are at, or near, capacity and all existing national cemeteries are expected to be full by the year 2020. The cemeteries that are full, however, can still accept cremation burials or inurnment of cremains in columbaria. The NCS states that efforts are under way to acquire additional cemetery lands, adjacent to existing national cemeteries whenever possible.

One of the things of which veterans should be aware is that a burial site cannot be reserved. You can't even apply for a site until the time of death. I imagine it would be quite disconcerting to a family to learn that the national cemetery closest to their home might already be full and their loved one might, instead, be interred hundreds of miles away. This potential problem can be compounded by overcrowding so that a spouse or other family members might not be buried next to the veteran.

Interment in a national cemetery is available to all members and veterans (if not dishonorably discharged) of the United States armed forces; spouses; widows and widowers who did not remarry; minor children; and—

under certain conditions—unmarried adult children. Also eligible are members of the armed forces reserves who die while on active duty and training for, or performing in, the duties of the reserves, or who have 20 years of service in the reserves.

While the NCS does not arrange for the funerals, it does offer a wide range of benefits at taxpayers' expense including the opening and closing of the grave sites. Also provided are headstones or markers. These markers can be flat (made of bronze, granite, or marble) or upright (made of granite or marble). The markers are inscribed with the name of the deceased, dates of birth and death, and branch of military service.

If the person is to be buried in a cemetery other than a national, military post, or state veterans' cemetery, the headstone or marker must be applied for through the United States Department of Veterans Affairs (VA)—formerly known as the Veterans Administration. In such instances, the headstone or marker will be shipped at government expense but the family must pay the cost of installation.

The VA will pay eligible recipients up to a $1,500 burial allowance if the veteran's death is service-related, and will pay the cost of shipping the remains to the national cemetery nearest the veteran's home. The VA will pay $300 for funeral and burial expenses for those veterans who were eligible to receive pension or compensation at the time of death. Also, the VA will pay $150 for a burial plot when the veteran is not buried in a cemetery that's under the jurisdiction of the United States government. I don't know how the government arrived at these figures (then, again, I rarely understand how the government works), but $300 for funeral and burial expenses won't pay for very much at all, and the $150 burial plot allowance is but a fourth of the average cost for a grave site.

My attitude may appear to be unpatriotic, but I assure you that is not the case. I simply believe that the government should not be in competition with private businesses. It would be far more efficient and equitable, in my opinion, for the government to provide veterans' families with adequate financial reimbursement and allow them to select the services and the grave sites from private sources.

Graveyard Economics

Once you realize the basic numbers behind operating a cemetery, you might even be tempted to start your own! Hey, a lot of people have made a lot of money doing just that.

First, consider that you can squeeze approximately 1,000 adult-sized graves into just one acre of land. Occasionally, two caskets are buried in the same grave— being buried in the same grave as a loved one is requested more often than you may realize, and some graves are even "triples." Also, a separate part of the cemetery is frequently used for the graves of infants and the number of these graves per acre is obviously much higher than for adults. But, for the sake of simplicity, we'll base our calculations on burying 1,000 adult bodies, one to a grave.

Using actual figures from one of my own operations, grave sites could range from $95 to $1,200, depending upon location—hilltops being more favorable and, therefore, more expensive, than bottomlands that would occasionally flood during heavy rains. The average, though, was about $600. Multiply that times the 1,000 sites and, just for the graves, we could realize $600,000. With the average purchase price of $2,000 per acre of land, that yields a gross profit per acre of $598,000.

That profit, of course, is just for the land. We would also factor in another $1,600 per plot (i.e., $500 for a vault, $600 for opening and closing the grave, and $500 for an average memorial) for a total of $2,200 for each of the plots. That increased our take to $2.2 million!

Mausoleums, of course, are even more space-efficient. The 1,000 caskets could be placed in a single building occupying less than one-third the square footage required to bury them in the ground. In one of our typical community-type mausoleums, we had 1,500 crypts. These varied in price from $900 to $3,000, depending again upon placement. That's right, "location-location-location," just as in real estate—which, in a sense, is just what this is.

The average crypt sold for $1,800. Multiply that times 1,500 crypts and, just for the crypts, we could realize $2.7 million. An average mausoleum costs $750,000 to construct, including a special ventilation system to exhaust any escaping odors of decomposition. The gross profit on this typical mausoleum was nearly $2 million.

In a columbarium, the percentage of profit is equally impressive. In a wall structure, we could have spaces for 100 urns. These niches would sell for an average $400 each (within a range of $200 to $900, again depending upon the location selected). According to my records, the construction of that wall columbarium probably cost us $6,000, for a gross profit of $34,000.

Before you rush out and start marking off potential grave sites in your backyard, beware there are unavoidable costs associated with cemetery management. It's not easy to find good sales people to sell the lots and you have to pay them high commissions to work for you. Also, before your calculator cools off, you must factor in the time element. When you open your gates, customers are not going to stream in to bury their dead. It may take 10 years or more before all the grave sites are sold and the money is yours.

Opening/Closing Graves and Other Costs

The figures shown in the examples above, however, are just the beginning of the story. Cemetery operators have quite a few other ways of jacking up the final bill to the consumer. The prices charged for opening and closing the grave site lead the way. ˙

In times past, graves were routinely dug by hand. Well-muscled grave diggers could open a grave in under two hours, longer if the ground was rocky or frozen. Today, of course, the operation is mechanized. A backhoe operator can open a grave in less than 30 minutes, and close it in even less time.

So what are the charges for this prodigious output of labor? The average cost to cemetery operators in the United States for digging and filling in a grave can run from $50 to $75, depending primarily on soil conditions. The charge to the customer, however, is normally $300 to $400 (some East Coast cemeteries charge as much as $1,500), and there's been a recent push in the industry to raise the average to $600 to $700. You can usually expect to pay more—frequently double overtime—if the grave is opened or closed on evenings, weekends, or holidays.

DON'T PLACE YOUR TRUST IN ANTI-TRUST

There is a legislative movement under way to pass state laws that would make cemeteries the only entities empowered to open and close graves. I should know—I was an integral part of that movement.

In 1993, I was serving as a member of a legislative subcommittee of the West Virginia Cemetery Association. The subcommittee was drafting a proposed bill for the state legislature that dealt with the trusting of funds from the sale of pre-need vaults. When we finished our draft legislation, we sent it to the American Cemetery Association (*note*: the ACA has since changed its name to the International Cemetery and Funeral Association) for its legal review. As part of its recommendation, the association added a section that would make it illegal for anyone other than a cemetery to open and close graves in the state of West Virginia. We submitted the bill to the legislature which passed it into law without ever questioning that rather dubious provision.

There have been legal actions in recent years attempting to prove the existence of collusion among cemeteries to maintain artificially high prices for the simple process of opening and closing graves. These actions, however, were settled out of court and the records were sealed. I remain convinced, however, that tying the sale of a cemetery plot to the requirement that only the cemetery be empowered to open and close the grave is a violation of antitrust laws. Perhaps, in time, a consumer lawsuit will prevail in this regard.

And don't forget to add in the cost and installation of the grave vault or liner.

As mentioned earlier, a concrete grave liner can cost anywhere from $200 to $400 and a vault from $300 to $10,000. If we sold the liner or the vault, the cost of the labor to place the liner or vault in the grave was included in the purchase price. If they were purchased elsewhere, we would charge $50 for the labor to install a liner and $75 to install a vault.

Perhaps because of a spirit of economy and a compelling need to feel even closer to the deceased, you'd like to gather some of your friends and dig the grave yourself. Maybe you're fortunate and even have a buddy who owns a backhoe. To my knowledge, there are still few laws or governmental regulations preventing such a noble endeavor. The cemetery, however, is ready for you on this one. They will no doubt require the posting of a performance bond, evidence of more than ample liability insurance, and probably more. These requirements are particularly distressing since their sole purpose is to maintain the cemeteries as the sole providers of these services. Therefore, you should be aware though, that it is quite common for the cemetery professionals themselves, when opening and closing graves, to damage an adjacent grave. Backhoes frequently dig too close to the adjoining grave site and crack or otherwise damage the vault. In rocky areas, dynamite may be required to blast before digging, and the explosions frequently crack vaults and caskets that might be nearby. The cemeteries merely cover up the damage, and the families are usually none the wiser.

OPEN GRAVE

A grave is not six feet deep, as is commonly believed. Most graves are four to five feet deep (and three and one-half feet wide, and eight feet long). By the time the cover to the liner or vault is in place, only about 12 to18 inches of dirt separate your feet from the top of the vault. Before digging the grave, the grass is removed in strips and set aside to be replaced when the grave is filled in. The dirt that is removed is either trucked away from the site, or left nearby and usually covered with a blanket of artificial grass.

After the grave is dug and the liner or vault placed in the hole, a lowering device—that's the shiny metal thing with wide canvas straps that you've seen holding the coffin suspended above the hole during the graveside service—is moved into place.

Once the mourners leave, the coffin is lowered into the grave, the liner or vault lid is installed securely in place, and the grave diggers begin shoveling (a backhoe is often used) the dirt back into the grave, compacting the dirt as they go to help prevent any settling of the earth. The pneumatic-powered soil tamping equipment frequently cracks the lid and seals of the vaults, rendering them almost immediately useless for the purpose of protecting the casketed body and grave for which they were sold.

A Grave Business Opportunity

There still remains in most states, though, a very lucrative business opportunity. Professional excavators, accustomed to the types of legal and financial requirements imposed by the cemeteries, could open and close graves at a considerable savings to consumers and yet realize an appreciable profit. When excavation equipment broke down at our cemeteries, we would turn to an outside contractor to come in and do the job. The typical fee we were charged was $125, and the excavator was making a profit. Perhaps, in the future, this will become more common.

As an aside, did you ever wonder why the casket is seldom lowered into the grave and the grave filled in while the mourners are still present? Most believe it is because it is too dramatic a scene for the bereaved to be emotionally capable of handling. Too often that is actually the case, as the process does not always go smoothly. I have witnessed interments where the lowering devices got stuck and the casket had to be wrestled into the ground. I've seen others where the straps holding the casket have snapped causing the casket to dangle over the open grave. And the number of times I've seen grave diggers slip and fall into the grave while filling it in are too numerous to count. So it's probably true that it is too dramatic a scene for the bereaved to be able to handle! I don't know who Murphy (of Murphy's Law fame) was, but I'm convinced he worked for a cemetery.

Memorial gardens have snatched the sale of grave markers away from the old guard monument makers. By dictating through their rules and regulations that all graves must be marked by particular type of bronze marker (they frequently specify not only the shape and size, but also the exact metal alloy content), and by setting themselves up as the only possible provider of such "acceptable" markers, memorial gardens have succeeded in reserving these profits entirely for themselves. You can expect to pay anywhere from $450 to $10,000 for a grave marker, usually cast in bronze, to mark a grave site in a memorial garden.

But by now you know it doesn't stop there, don't you? Of course it doesn't. The cemetery's charge for the labor necessary to install the marker on the grave is included in the purchase price. If you purchased a marker elsewhere that was acceptable to the cemetery, the cemetery will charge you at least $ .25 to $ .40 per square inch to install it.

A SIGN OF THE TIMES?

From the Charleston, West Virginia *Gazette* (February 6, 1996) comes this story:

In March 1995, a Jumping Branch, West Virginia, woman prematurely gave birth to twin boys. They died one day later, and they were buried in Restwood Cemetery near the town of Hinton.

A full year later, their double grave remained unmarked. The grandfather refuses to pay the cemetery the $500 it demands for installing the marker. (Note: Installing a marker is similar to installing a piece of paving stone in a yard—make a shallow hole the size of the stone, level out the bottom, pour in some gravel, level it off again, and place the stone.)

A major consolidator had purchased the cemetery in 1994, along with 11 others in the state and promptly raised prices (opening and closing a grave there now costs $495 before 3:00 p.m. and $595 after 3:00 p.m. on weekdays, $895 on Sundays, and $995 on legal holidays).

The grandfather is angry because he feels there are no other options available to him in the area. The chairman of the Cemetery Consumers Service Council for the state cemetery association—himself an owner of a cemetery—countered, "You can't monopolize the cemetery industry in a state where you can bury someone in your backyard."

The *Gazette* reported that the cemetery will allow the grandfather to bring in an outside contractor, provided it is a reputable firm with a long history. Even if such a firm were found to be acceptable to the cemetery, the grandfather said, the cemetery would no doubt charge him a fee for a cemetery employee to watch the installation to make certain the job was done properly. He assumes, and probably rightly so, that the total bill would be at least equal to the $500 the cemetery wants to charge him.

Meanwhile, his grandsons' grave marker remains covered by a piece of felt in his garage.

If your loved one is being interred in a cemetery that allows monuments, the cemetery will attempt to sell you this type of marker as well. You are not restricted, however, in this regard and are free to purchase it from an outside monument maker; although there will, no doubt, be cemetery restrictions as to size and style. And, as with the memorial garden markers, be prepared to pay the cemetery's labor rate for the installation of the monument you purchase elsewhere.

CEMETERY RULES AND REGULATIONS

Anytime you buy a lot in a cemetery, you are agreeing to abide by the cemetery's rules and regulations. Though they are important, the consumer seldom reads them. Typically, they are in very fine print and laced with legalese. As they are a part of the contract, take the time to read them before signing it. This is a *very* long-term purchase you're making here!

The cost of *perpetual care* of the grave site is contained within the purchase price of the lot. This cost is to cover the landscape maintenance (i.e., mowing, weeding, trimming, and removal of flowers and leaves, etc.)—perpetually. Be aware, however, that perpetual care does not cover the grave marker. In most instances, the marker is covered by the person's homeowner's insurance policy.

Non-Profit Does NOT = No Profits

Few cemeteries pay property taxes, as taxing authorities rationalize that the land can never be commercially developed. To add to this tax break, many private cemeteries in the United States are organized as non-profit corporations. Lest you tend to lump all non-profit entities together with such organizations as the Boy Scouts of America or the United Way, please read on.

While the operator can somewhat justifiably contend that the cemetery provides a needed and worthwhile service to the community, it does so frequently at tremendous and untaxed profits. If it is organized as a non-profit corporation, the cemetery's revenues are not subject to federal, state, or local taxes. It's entirely legal.

How does it work? A non-profit cemetery usually does not own the land itself. Rather, the land is frequently owned by a separate entity—either by individuals or by a separate corporation controlled by them. These individuals or their corporation will contract with the non-profit cemetery corporation (also run by the same individuals in most instances) to sell grave sites and manage the cemetery.

These individuals or their corporation will receive, for example, up to 90% of the revenues received from the sale of grave sites, mausoleum crypts, and columbaria niches. The non-profit cemetery will pay for all landscape and maintenance costs and all other general operating expenses out of the remaining 10%.

6

Ding-Dong... Cemetery Calling!

Door-to-Door Death Sales

"We simply rob ourselves when we make presents to the dead."
Publilius Syrus, *Moral Sayings* (1st Century B.C.)
[1034 translation, Drius Lyman}

The Avon lady doesn't come to the door anymore and neither does the Fuller Brush man. In what must be one of the last bastions of door-to-door selling, cemetery plot salespeople ply their trade with continued fervor. I personally believe the whole industry is at least 20 to 30 years behind current marketing trends, but cemeterians remain convinced the only effective way to sell is to get into the consumer's home. The vast majority of cemetery salespersons I've known are poorly trained fast talkers who get in, sell, and get out as quickly as they can. If your doorway has never been graced by one of these folks, relax...it's only a matter of time.

For the most part, they are nice enough folks and I have a lot of respect for them as individuals. Their employers are the ones I hold responsible for leading them down the path of deceptive practices.

Some cemeteries have sales forces of literally thousands of these representatives who descend upon neighborhoods at dusk. These sales folks are amazingly effective. This is how I started—this is where I first learned the business.

You are too sophisticated, you say? Too worldly to buy anything from a door-to-door salesperson, especially something so serious as a cemetery plot? Perhaps so. But there must be millions of others unlike you, for these sales-people rack up millions of dollars in sales each year. But just in case you might feel even a little bit vulnerable were one of them to call on you, let me share some typical presentation techniques. These are some of the things I personally did, and they are the things many sales representatives are taught to do.

There Ain't No Such Thing as a *Free* Lot

Cemeteries employ many sales gimmicks. One fairly common ploy is to offer a "free lot" to just about anybody, but particularly members of groups (e.g., veterans organizations, associations for senior citizens, Rotary Club, Elks, etc.). The hidden purpose, of course, is to lock the recipient and his family in as the cemetery's customers. But there are no free lots for these relatives, so the recipient will have to buy additional spaces. Not surprisingly, the so-called "free lots" are usually in the least desirable sections of the cemetery.

But is a "free lot" really free? Hardly. The recipient of this "gift" will be required to pay perpetual care, the cost of opening and closing the grave, and frequently have to remit a yearly or semiannual fee to maintain the lot on the records. If the recipient fails to pay, the lot will revert back to the cemetery.

Other Tricks of the Trade

Our cemetery offered top-of-the-line services and products, and our costs were priced accordingly. Our salespeople were indoctrinated to believe that the consumer was willing to pay more money because we offered quality. We convinced our people that every door they knocked on had a $100 bill on the other side of it. All they had to do was get inside the home and make sure that they got it. It was either the customer's $100 bill or theirs. Not surprisingly, they felt they needed it more than the consumer did.

Once inside the home, our salespeople would frequently be confronted with a consumer who wanted to be cremated. They were trained to answer, "Would you really be able to cremate one of your children?!" While people tended to be callous when discussing their own eventual demise, bringing children into the presentation generally softened them up a great deal.

Actually, it really didn't matter what they said they wanted to buy. We sold what we wanted and were told to sell, and we used every sales technique to make certain we were successful. We would do things so crass as actually pretending to be hard of hearing when the consumer voiced an objection. Some of our sales representatives even went so far as to wear fake hearing aids as props. If a customer raised a particularly strong objection to the presentation, the salesperson would begin adjusting the hearing device and just smile blankly at the customer and pretend they never heard the objection. We were masters of manipulation and consistently sold to between 35% to 40% of all the people upon whom we called.

Interestingly, the vast majority of our customers were in the lower to middle socio-economic levels of the community. By contrast, we had quite a difficult time even getting into the homes of the more educated, more affluent people who were generally disinclined to purchase anything from door-to-door salespeople. Demographics, therefore, played a big part when we mapped out our marketing strategies. My experience is borne out by a market research study commissioned by the funeral and cemetery industries (*1995 Study of American Attitudes Toward Ritualization and Memorialization*, prepared by The Wirthlin Group, of McLean, Virginia). The report reveals that individuals earning less than $30,000 per year are significantly more likely than those earning over $50,000 a year to prearrange.

BLUE SUEDE SHOES WALKIN' THROUGH THOSE TALL DOORS

We frequently, and derogatorily, referred to the affluent as "tall doors" since their homes were often quite impressive and many actually seemed to have taller doors! In all fairness, though, our high-pressure salespeople were often described equally derogatorily as "blue suede shoes."

Discounts are routinely offered while the sales representative is in the customer's home. Customers are told that this is the only time the discount would be available. For instance, customers might be told that a cemetery package, regularly priced at $1,500, could be purchased for the discounted price of $1,300—but only if the customer bought it immediately, right there on the spot. Frequently, this isn't true, of course. The customer could walk into the cemetery's offices the next day and purchase the very same package at its regular price of $1,300. They get away with it simply because no one ever comes into the office to check.

Another typical sales trick is to take a spouse "out of the picture" during the presentation. We would say, for example, "Mrs. Jones, let's just pretend for a moment that Mr. Jones is dead. What would you be doing right now if he were dead?"

Then we would be silent for a few moments and watch her reaction. We would then proceed to tell her what she'd be doing: making funeral arrangements, making burial arrangements, calling family members and friends, and handling all the other things that must be done when a death occurs.

Hopefully having shocked them at the enormity and complexity of post-death responsibilities, we would continue, "All these are things that *must* be done. Wouldn't it be far simpler if you and Mr. Jones, in the reasonableness of the present moment, made these decisions tonight? Wouldn't it be more comforting to do so together, without one of you being deceased? Wouldn't it make a lot more sense than putting if off until Mr. Jones is gone and you're wondering what he may have wanted?

111

Did he want to be buried on a hilltop? What kind of a casket would he have wanted?"

Our success relied heavily on getting the consumers emotionally involved in the conversation. Frequently, the husband or wife (or, ideally, both) would cry while we were completing our sales pitch. That was absolutely wonderful as far as we were concerned, as tears meant we'd probably be able to close the sale right then and there.

The Five Emotions of Buying

Our salespeople were trained to probe for one of the five basic emotions that would prove to be the customer's motivating reason for buying: love, fear, need, greed, and desire. One of these would prove to be the "hot button" for the consumer and it was our job to find it and zero in on it.

If *love* were the controlling emotion, we made certain we spoke often of love during the presentation. We'd say it was obvious how much the husband and wife loved each other and we'd stress how truly loving it is to arrive at these decisions together on a pre-need basis.

We could use the emotion of *need* if the consumer had lost a loved one and not yet made arrangements to be buried next to that person.

Greed was presumed to be the motivating factor if we determined that the family was concerned about cost. In this instance, we stressed the in-home discount angle. We made certain they understood that buying that very night was the only way they were going to be able to take advantage of the reduced price we were offering and to have a chance at avoiding future inflation.

If the *desire* to have the finest things in life proved to be important, then we were the company for them. As I mentioned, we were a high-end company, tops in products and services, and certainly tops in price. We appealed openly to their need for purchasing only the very best.

Fear was the easy one! If we sensed a consumer was afraid to make funeral and burial arrangements without the spouse present, we pulled out all stops and literally scared them into making the decision.

If a client objected to our prices, our standard reply was, "Yes, I agree. They are high. On the other hand, can you honestly say you can afford to settle for less?" Then we would focus on the issue of buying right then and there, thereby locking in the price and protecting the purchase from the ravages of inflation.

Moving in for the Close

One of our favorite slogans was: *Customers buy on emotion and justify the purchase with logic.* We used the emotional sales pitch throughout the presentation and moved smoothly to the logic of the "Right Way—Wrong Way" close.

"Mr. and Mrs. Jones," we would say, "there is a right way and a wrong way to do everything. The right way is to do it right here and now while both of you are in a logical and unemotional state of mind and can make this rational decision together. The wrong way to make this decision is for one of you, on the very worst day of your life, to be forced to make these choices without knowing what your spouse wanted. Plus, there is a much greater financial risk in doing it later when one of you is alone.

Do you want to make this decision the right way or the wrong way?" Then we would employ the very effective tool of silence.

Of course, they wanted to do it the right way, but often they wanted to think it over and discuss it just between the two of them. Our scripted response would be, "You've been married how many years? During that time, how often have you actually talked about this subject?" They would usually confess they'd never even broached the subject. "Even if you have talked about this before, have you done anything about it? Obviously not, or we wouldn't be sitting here tonight talking about it again. What makes you think this time will be different? My guess is that if you don't make this decision now, you won't take any action. Then one of you will be forced into making these very same decisions on absolutely the worst day of your life. Again, which is better: to do it together now or for one of you to do it alone later?"

Occasionally, we'd encounter a curmudgeon who would say something such as, "I don't care what they do with me when I die. They can just throw me over the hill for all I care!" In response, we would look at the wife and say, "Well, Mrs. Smith, could you throw your husband's body over the hill?" Or we might turn to the husband and say, "How many children do you have, Mr. Smith? Can you honestly tell me you could throw one of them over the hill?" The responses were obviously different when the body was of a loved one than if they were just thinking of themselves.

Lest you think my salespeople and I were simply evil mavericks preying alone on the unsuspecting customers, let me share with you some excerpts from the *Sales Meetings Guidebook* published in an article in the

February 1996 issue of *Cemetery Management*. About the importance of product knowledge versus closing techniques, the article said, "Our attitude in closing is more important than our aptitude in product knowledge..." The emphasis on the emotional involvement of the consumer is evident as the article states, "In our presentation, we must 'back the hearse up to smell the flowers.' There are many ways to do this, but one of the most effective ways is to remove the husband from the picture and take the widow on a death shopping spree."

Wherefore Art Thou, Consumer?

I must confess I don't recall any discussion at our sales meetings about serving the needs of the consumer. All we ever talked about was sell—sell—sell. We stressed how important it was that the representatives concentrate on selling the more expensive items. That would benefit the company, of course, but it would also benefit the sales-people who worked on commission.

Most cemetery salespeople receive very little training. Most are hired on the "warm body" theory (i.e., anybody who has a warm body and a car is qualified to sell cemetery plots and merchandise). There are many sales managers working for some of the largest cemetery operations in the country who take great pride in bragging about how quickly they can get newly hired counselors into the field selling. The practice is to hire someone, offer some minimal training, and put the person in the field quickly and see whether that person sinks or swims.

I found it takes a salesperson about six months to develop a true understanding of the products and services. Yet, we placed these people in the customers' homes to sell some of the most important purchases one will ever make—and this after one or two days of classroom training in selling and closing techniques, and not on product knowledge.

I've already confessed that I'm no saint. I ran a cemetery sales force the same as I just described. Further, I have participated in many national industry forums and training seminars in order to help spread this type of sales knowledge far and wide. Speaking on my own behalf, however, I want to add that I tried unsuccessfully for years to get the cemetery business to alter its sales approach. Unfortunately, many of the leaders matured in the industry decades ago and refuse to change how they market their products. Quite frankly, I am amazed at my own success and at the continued success of the industry—a success that can be attributed to "hot" salespeople and to a buying public sadly lacking the information which would enable them to make wise purchase decisions.

A couple of years ago, a personal acquaintance—one of the top executives in one of the largest public cemetery operations in the country—told me, "There is still only one way to sell cemetery lots and that is to knock on a door unexpectedly and walk in and close the sale." He said he didn't believe in making sales appointments nor did he believe you should tell the family at the outset who you are or what you want. One of the tactics he used (and is also used in every state where cemeteries can get away with it) was to knock on the door of the unsuspecting consumer and say, "Good evening, Mrs. Jones, may I come in?" Even in today's climate of high crime and scare-tactic headlines, you'd be absolutely astounded at how often this ploy works.

Is There a Better Way?

Though the cemeteries are reluctant to change their sales strategies, I believe that with a shift in marketing focus the consumer could be enticed to come into the cemetery office and purchase. The consumer, though, must first be told about the available products and their prices. The buying public needs to be made aware of the advantages of making the purchases and be presented with honestly priced choices.

If cemeteries eliminated the high-commission salespeople and spent half of the commission money on advertising, they could then use the other half to reduce their inflated prices. I am convinced that, if they were to do so, the public would come in and buy. Even though the cemeteries would make the same amount of money and probably more, it's not likely to happen. Meanwhile, the industry stubbornly continues along with its marketing blinders in place, as the following story will show.

At a 1995 convention of cemeterians, there was an hour-long sales panel session that provided the audience with "hot tips" designed to increase sales production. The panel, comprised of 12 industry sales managers who represented a total of 6,000 sales representatives (one, a sales executive with a large conglomerate based in Houston, Texas, was himself responsible for 3,800 sales-people, and another represented 171 cemeteries—I'm telling you, this is *big* business, folks) delivered one-minute suggestions over the background music of Johnny

Carson's *Tonight Show* theme song. None of the tips ever mentioned product quality, customer service, or the needs of the consumer. Instead, there were the usual ideas such as bonuses, tropical vacations, and luxury automobiles to spur sales performance. Here is a sampling of some of the other ideas given the audience:

• One executive said he labeled the back wall of his cemetery's salesroom the "Wall of Shame" and he placed there the names of salespeople whose production fell below their assigned quotas. He labeled the front wall the "The Wall of Fame" and listed there the names of those who met or exceeded their goals. Humiliation is a great motivator, he suggested.

• One sales manager challenged his representatives to a contest. If they, as a group, beat their sales quotas for a month, he said he would sit on top of the cemetery's mausoleum for an entire day. They did and he did (conjures up quite a picture of dignity and solemnity, doesn't it?).

• Another speaker bemoaned the low turnout of veterans when he had tried to lure them onto his cemetery property for Memorial Day observances and sales pitches. He came up with the idea he unabashedly called his "Buy A Veteran Program." In a circular mailed to veterans prior to Memorial Day one year, he offered them silver coins if they showed up. The attendance was great, he said, and the next year he offered them a framed set of coins minted during World War II.

• The kitchen table is where the grave sites should be sold as the kitchen table forces eye contact, said another. Besides, he added, the kitchen table is the inner sanctum of the home—the place where important family decisions are made.

• Feign concern for neighborhood safety as a means of making additional appointments, suggested another sales manager. He tells his salespeople to arrive 15 minutes early for a scheduled appointment, then go to the home across the street and introduce themselves. Express support of neighborhood crime watches, they're taught to say. Tell the neighbors you're in the neighborhood to meet with the Joneses and you didn't want your "strange" car to be of concern to them; and then try to set an appointment.

• Perhaps one of the most revealing suggestions was to take "at least one dollar down" on a pre-need contract if the salesperson was unable to close the entire deal. That way, the audience was told, the customer is locked into the prices offered for one year and can be reapproached in 12 months and a new sales attempt made. If the customer died during the year and a funeral director called to make arrangements, the cemetery was in a position (with just that one dollar down) to say that the family had already made their purchase.

This was a high-powered panel of the most accomplished salespeople in the nation speaking to an audience of those who aspired to emulate them. Is it any wonder that change is so long in coming to the death merchants?

7

Congress and the Corpse

Government Takes a Grave Interest in the Business

"Laws are like cobwebs, which may catch small flies, but let wasps and hornets break through."

Jonathan Swift,
A Critical Essay upon the Faculties of the Mind (1707)

The death merchants complain loudly—as do many other types of businesses—about the amount of government interference in their daily lives. There are numerous federal, state, and local laws and agencies governing the funeral and cemetery industries, among them the Occupational Safety and Health Administration (OSHA), the Environmental Protection Agency (EPA), and the Federal Trade Commission (FTC).

The FTC Adopts the Funeral Rule

Jessica Mitford, who wrote the book *The American Way of Death* (1963, Simon and Schuster), is given credit by many for providing Congress with the impetus to do something about the abuses that were running rampant throughout the funeral industry even at that time. As a result of this and other similar outcries, Congress thoroughly investigated the industry during nearly two years of hearings that began in the early 1980s. The hearings eventually resulted in the promulgation by the FTC of the Funeral Industry Practices Rule (Funeral Rule) [Appendix I].

The legislative intent of the Funeral Rule, adopted in 1984, was to regulate funeral homes and to ensure that consumers would be given the information necessary to make informed decisions before making funeral arrangements. An ancillary benefit, both legislators and industry reformers hoped, would be to curb the spiraling costs of funerals and burials.

As is often the case with such instances of originally good legislative intent, the results were disappointing. Cemeterians spent hundreds of thousands of dollars in lobbying efforts that proved successful in keeping their industry entirely out of the FTC's recommendations. For its part, the National Funeral Directors Association (NFDA) proudly stated that it lobbied long and hard during the hearings and boasted it convinced the FTC to delete several consumer protection clauses from the Funeral Rule before it was approved. Among the sections the NFDA apparently found too onerous for inclusion were:

• A stipulation that funeral homes display three of their cheapest caskets.

• That funeral directors must explain that burial vaults and liners may also be purchased at cemeteries.

• Provide consumers, upon request, explanations—in writing—of any law necessitating the purchase of any merchandise or service.

• Pass along to consumers any rebates, commission, or volume discounts the funeral home might receive.

Even with these so-called victories, the death merchants continued their struggle, fighting legal battles and mounting massive lobbying efforts to get the Funeral Rule abolished. As the FTC held more hearings in recent years to fine tune the Funeral Rule, it waded through numerous federal and private industry surveys and heard dozens upon dozens of industry proponents and opponents to the regulations. Among those arguing for the abolition of the Funeral Rule, not surprisingly, were the NFDA and the National Concrete Burial Vault Association. They contended that the Funeral Rule was simply unnecessary at best, and an unfair imposition of burdensome administrative costs at worst.

Fortunately for consumers, the FTC discovered in its surveys that industry compliance with the Funeral Rule was woefully lacking and found the testimony of opponents to be specious. In the end and to its credit, the FTC ignored the whining and ranting of the industry's wily rascals and made some minor modifications in amending the Funeral Rule in January 1994.

You can skip the fine-print, legal mumbo-jumbo of the appendices to this book if you wish, but I do want to point out some aspects of the Funeral Rule with which you should be familiar to help you be a more informed consumer.

Letting Your Fingers Do the Walking

The cornerstone of the Funeral Rule is the regulation requiring funeral directors to provide consumers with specific and detailed price information in advance so that the consumers can then purchase only the funeral merchandise and funeral services that they desire. When a consumer phones a funeral provider and inquires about terms, conditions, or prices of funeral goods or services, the funeral provider is required to:

1. Give the consumer the prices and any other information from price lists to help answer the questions.

2. Give the consumer any other information about prices or offerings that is readily available and reasonably answers the consumer's questions.

The intent is to enable consumers to comparison-shop by telephone before selecting the funeral home, goods, and services.

Information for the Consumer

GENERAL PRICE LIST—The GPL [Appendix II] is a written list that must clearly identify and itemize prices for all the goods and services (e.g., embalming, service fees, cash advance items, cremation caskets, and required purchases) that a funeral director provides.

Funeral directors are required to give their GPL to anyone who asks in person about funeral goods, funeral services, or their prices. The request does not have to come from someone wishing to arrange a funeral; the GPL must be given to *anyone* who requests it, including journalists, religious groups, consumer organizations, etc. The GPL is to be given to the person to keep. The Funeral Rule, however, does not require a funeral director to mail out the GPL to someone who may call on the phone or write and inquire about prices.

The funeral director may not insist that callers give their names, addresses, or phone numbers as a prerequisite for answering their questions, and the funeral director may not require the callers to come in person to the funeral homes to get price information. If those making the calls or writing the letters of inquiry show up at the funeral homes, the funeral director is required, at that point, to provide them with the GPL.

The FTC says the GPL must be presented when any discussion begins about the type of funeral or disposition that may be arranged, the specific goods and services that are offered, or the prices of those goods and services. Also, the face-to-face contact that makes it necessary to give out the GPL does not have to occur in the funeral home. It can happen anywhere (e.g., private home, hospital, nursing facility, etc.), but the GPL is not required to be given if the funeral home staff is only removing the body to the funeral home and does not engage in any discussion of goods, services, or prices.

The FTC discovered in its investigation of levels of compliance with the Funeral Rule that many funeral homes were simply showing the GPL to consumers and not actually giving it to them. The law specifically requires that each consumer receive a written copy of the GPL to keep and, though you would hope this admonition was unnecessary, the FTC warns funeral directors that they may not charge the customer for the GPL.

Anyone (other than a cemetery) who is selling funeral/burial goods and services on a pre-need basis is covered by the Funeral Rule and are, therefore, required to give the consumer the GPL.

The FTC suggests that the GPL be either typewritten or printed (be especially wary, I presume, if the GPL you receive is written in crayon!). The GPL must include the name, address, and telephone number of the funeral provider's place of business, the effective date of the GPL, and be captioned "General Price List."

To better enable consumers to select only those goods and services they desire, the items listed below must be included, along with their corresponding individual prices, on the GPL:

Forwarding of Remains to, and Receiving Remains from, Another Funeral Home— The GPL should contain one price for each of these items and it should clearly explain all the services that will be performed for the quoted price. Further, the prices should include all charges related to each service. Any pricing method is acceptable (flat fee, hourly fee, mileage fee, etc.), as long as it clearly disclosed.

Direct Cremations—The GPL must quote a price range for direct cremations, and must be accompanied by the disclosure language about the availability of alternative containers. The GPL must also include the following options within the price range: one price in instances where the casket or alternative container is provided by the consumer, and a separate price when the funeral home provides the alternative container. The Funeral Rule specifically requires that alternative containers be made available when direct cremations are provided. If the cremation will be provided by an outside crematory, the customer should be advised that there will be an additional charge added by that crematory to the consumer's bill.

Immediate Burials—The GPL must include one price for immediate burials in which the casket is provided by the consumer and a separate price when the funeral home provides the casket or alternative container. Information detailing the services and the containers must also be included.

Basic Services of Funeral Director and Staff (and Overhead)—This non-declinable fee can include charges for all services provided by a funeral home—from storing the remains to arranging and providing the funeral. The basic services fee cannot include any charges for items that the consumer may decline and must be, by law, listed separately on the GPL. Overhead expenses (e.g., salaries, taxes, insurance, fees, etc.) can be included in the basic services fee, or allocated to the goods and services provided, or a combination of the two, but overhead cannot be charged separately elsewhere. The FTC's Funeral Rule clearly states that the basic services fee is the *only* non-declinable fee permitted (unless state or local law requires otherwise). The industry had begun to charge other non-declinable fees for such things as "basic utilities" and "casket handling." Any non-declinable fee, other than the basic services fee, is in violation of the law.

This is all well and good, but can you name any other industry that is authorized by the federal government to charge consumers for overhead and profit as a prerequisite for doing business? *Consumers Digest* (September/October 1995) quoted Lisa Carlson, of the Memorial Society of Vermont, as reporting to the FTC that the average basic services fees had escalated approximately 80% since the FTC incorporated the fee in its regulations.

Embalming—The price must include all charges for the preparation room, professional services, equipment, and materials. An embalming fee can only be charged if (1) state or local law requires embalming under the circumstances involving a particular body; (2) prior approval has been obtained from the family or another authorized person; or (3) *all* of the following apply: the funeral director is unable to contact the family or an authorized person, the funeral director has no reason to believe that the family does not want embalming, and approval is received subsequent to the embalming. If in this latter case, however, the body is embalmed and the family chooses a disposition not requiring an embalming, the funeral director cannot charge for the embalming.

Other Preparation of the Body—This fee is to include such things as cosmetic and restoration work. Also, if washing and disinfecting are used in lieu of embalming, these charges should be specified.

Use of Facilities and Staff for Viewing—Either a flat fee or an hourly rate may be charged the consumer for this item. The cost of facilities and staff should be included in one charge unless, of course, the viewing was held off-premises, in which case there should be no charge for facilities.

Use of Facilities and Staff for Funeral Ceremony or Memorial Service—Similarly, there should be one charge for facilities and staff if either the funeral ceremony or the memorial service is held at the funeral home. There should only be a charge for staff for funerals held at another location.

Use of Equipment and Staff for Graveside Service—This charge is intended for those instances in which the funeral service is held at the graveside and is not meant to include the briefer committal service that follows a funeral held elsewhere. This charge can include, for example, the cost of staff and equipment such as tents and chairs.

Hearse and Limousine—As with the transferring of remains, the funeral home may charge for the hearse on any basis it chooses—flat fee, hourly, mileage, etc. The FTC recognizes the occasional need for discounting prices (e.g., for funerals for friends or relatives, or purely for business purposes). The FTC states, however, that none of the prices should be inflated in order to offer all or most of the funeral home's customers a discounted price. In that instance, according to the FTC, the discounted price is the actual price and should be so reflected on the GPL.

CASKET PRICE LIST—The CPL contains the prices of caskets [Appendix III]. The CPL must include the retail price of each casket and alternative container stocked by the funeral home. The CPL must include information sufficient to identify each available casket (e.g., gauge of metal or type of wood, exterior trim, interior fabric, etc.).

A photograph or model number alone does not satisfy the requirements of law.

The funeral director must show the CPL to anyone who, in person, requests information about caskets and their prices. The law clearly states that the CPL must be shown to the consumer *before* being shown any caskets (any person who wants to change the selection of a casket purchased under a pre-need contract must also be shown the CPL). You will want to take your own notes, as the Funeral Rule does not require that copies of the CPL be given to the consumer to keep.

OUTER BURIAL CONTAINER PRICE LIST—The OBC contains the prices of outer burial containers [Appendix IV]. The OBC must include a complete description and the retail price of each outer burial container offered by the funeral home. The OBC must be shown to anyone requesting information about outer burial containers and prior to showing any such containers. As with the CPL, the funeral home is not required to give consumers a copy to keep.

STATEMENT OF FUNERAL GOODS AND SERVICES SELECTED—The Statement [Appendix V] is the itemized list of all the goods and services (and their prices) that the consumer has selected. It is illegal for the funeral director to aggregate costs on the Statement that are listed separately on the GPL. It provides the consumer with the detailed information necessary— including any legal, cemetery, or crematory requirements that require the purchase of any specific funeral goods or services—to review the decisions made and their corresponding costs.

The law requires the funeral director to give consumers the Statement at the end of the meeting in which the arrangements are made. It is a violation of the Funeral Rule to give the Statement to the consumer at the funeral or some other later date. If the arrangements were made over the telephone, it is incumbent upon the funeral director to get a copy of the Statement to the consumer at the very earliest possible opportunity.

Many funeral establishments, in response to the Funeral Rule, devised "funeral packages" as a way to avoid itemizing prices. While the FTC permits the use of package prices, they must be in addition to—and not in place of—the itemized prices required on the GPL. If a consumer selects a package, the Statement must describe the package and itemize and price each of the component goods and services of the package.

The Statement must also list separately each cash advance item. Cash advance items are those things secured from a third party and paid for by the funeral director on the customer's behalf (e.g., cemetery charges, pallbearers, public transportation, death certificates, obituaries, clergy honoraria, etc.). If the actual price of a cash advance item is not known ahead of time, the funeral home is required to enter an accurate estimate and provide the consumer with a written statement of the actual charge as soon as it is known.

Misrepresentation "No-No's"

The Funeral Rule specifically prohibits funeral directors from misrepresenting the following:

Embalming—Consumers must not be told that state or local laws require embalming when that is not the case. In fact, funeral directors are ordered to tell the consumer in writing that embalming is not required except in special circumstances. Again, state or local laws notwithstanding, it is illegal to tell a consumer that embalming is required for any reason when the consumer requests a direct cremation or burial, or when refrigeration is available and the consumer has selected a closed-casket service with no formal viewing.

Casket for Direct Cremation—Consumers must be told that no state or local laws require them to buy a casket for a direct cremation when there is no open-casket ceremony or viewing.

Outer Burial Container—It is illegal to tell consumers that state or local laws require the purchase of an outer burial container when that is not the case; nor can a funeral director tell a consumer that a particular cemetery requires an outer burial container when that is untrue.

Legal and Cemetery Requirements—It is illegal to tell consumers that any federal, state, or local laws (or any particular cemetery or crematory, for that matter) require them to purchase any specific goods or services when that is not the case. If there is such a law or requirement, the funeral director is required to identify and describe that law or requirement in writing to the consumer.

Preservative and Protective Value Claims—It is illegal to represent to consumers that funeral goods or services will delay the natural decomposition of human remains for either a long time or for an indefinite period. Further, it is illegal to tell consumers that such funeral goods as caskets and vaults possess protective features or will protect the body from grave-site substances. The funeral director is required by federal law to provide the consumer with all manufacturers' warranty information for goods the consumer has purchased.

Cash Advance Items—If the funeral director adds a charge to cash advance items or if the funeral director receives any kind of commission, discount, or rebate that is not passed on to the customer, the funeral director is prohibited from stating that the price charged on the Statement is the funeral director's cost. While federal law does not require the funeral director to disclose the amount of any commission, discount, or rebate, some state laws do.

Other Misrepresentations—Here's the catch-all phrase. The FTC prohibits any and all other mis-representations or deceptive practices not specifically prohibited by the Funeral Rule.

They Can't Just Make You Buy Stuff

The Funeral Rule prohibits the death merchants from forcing consumers to purchase goods and services that are unwanted and/or unneeded as a prerequisite for purchasing other goods and services they may desire. For example, this means it is illegal for a funeral director to charge an additional fee or a surcharge to consumers who might purchase a casket somewhere else. The FTC included this addition to the Funeral Rule, labeling such extra charges for casket handling as "simply a hidden penalty for those consumers who exercise the right to purchase a casket from another seller."

Also, a funeral director cannot alter prices based on the specific selections a consumer might make. The FTC explained, "Such a practice also would defeat the purpose of the Funeral Rule which is to give people accurate, itemized price information that affords them the opportunity to select the arrangements they want." The FTC does not require a funeral director to accommodate a consumer's requests if they are "impossible, impractical or excessively burdensome." Funeral directors, however, cannot refuse a request simply because they "don't like it or don't approve of it."

Both Enforcement and Compliance Are Spotty

Amazing as it may seem, the FTC's budget does not include any money for publicizing the Funeral Rule to the general public. It's a small wonder, then, that public awareness of the law and its provisions designed to protect us all is practically nonexistent.

There are approximately 22,000 funeral establishments in the United States handling more than two million funerals annually, yet there exists only a handful of FTC investigators to monitor them. As recently as 1995, only two FTC staff members were devoting a majority of their time to investigating possible violations of the commission's Funeral Rule. It's no surprise, then, that funeral directors continue to feel a sense of invulnerability.

Meanwhile, average funeral costs have continued to increase at a rate far exceeding the rate of inflation since the adoption of the Funeral Rule.

To beef up the efforts of its own staff, the FTC recently joined forces with state attorneys general in sporadic undercover sting operations that resulted in substantial fines to several funeral homes. In relatively few instances, however, has any of the money found its way back to the consumers who had been affected. The FTC reported that it discovered rates of noncompliance with the Funeral Rule ranging from 20% to 40%.

The NFDA is ever-vigilant, though, always looking for ways to come to the rescue of its poor, beleaguered members. The *Funeral Service Insider* newsletter (January 22, 1996) reported that the "FTC and NFDA are teaming up to take some of the pain out of FTC undercover Funeral Rule sting operations." This seemingly unlikely alliance of watchdog and wolf came up with the Funeral Rule Offenders Program (FROP).

FROP takes effect when a funeral home finds itself in the middle of an FTC investigation involving the itemized GPL (the program is expected to be expanded to include other types of alleged violations of the Funeral Rule, as well). The funeral home, with the FTC's blessing, has the option of letting the investigation continue (and run the risk of fines of up to $10,000 per violation) or paying a smaller fine (to be calculated at .008 times the firm's annual gross revenue for the past three fiscal years) and agreeing to participate in an NFDA-sponsored employee training program. If that weren't enough, the FTC has agreed to keep the names of the offending funeral homes a secret. Sweet deal! Think we could get the NFDA to arrange a similar escape route from the Internal Revenue Service for the rest of us? Not bloody likely.

The Wall Street Journal (January 11, 1996) reporting on FROP said, "To show contrition for failures to provide price lists to consumers, offenders would volunteer payments to the Treasury." The article added that the NFDA felt the program "would help offenders go straight."

In all my years in the business and in my involvement with several industry organizations, I've not seen a hint of contrition for anything from my colleagues. Make no mistake about it, this is as combative and defensive an industry as there is. The NFDA, apparently through high-pressure lobbying efforts, succeeded in undercutting the already limited enforcement power of the FTC.

The FTC appears to be enamored of the NFDA. The two are now cooperating on another new program: Consumer Assurance Program (CAP). CAP is supposed to be some sort of *Good Housekeeping* Seal of Approval for the funeral industry (I think I'll leave my doors unlocked at night, I feel so much safer now).

Warning to Consumers

Still, the Funeral Rule remains an important and potent piece of regulation. The mere fact that Congress found the rule necessary is evidence of the sorry state of affairs within the industry. That so many well-organized, financed, and powerful industry entities fought so hard against it (and continue to do so) lends even more credence to its importance.

The burden of ensuring compliance with the Funeral Rule unfortunately rests with the consumers since the

FTC, to a great extent, has abdicated that responsibility. The burden of becoming conversant with the Funeral Rule and how it can greatly assist in making informed decisions is also the public's responsibility. The FTC never really took it upon itself to inform the customer.

I realize that all this information about the Funeral Rule may appear tedious; but I urge you to reread it when you are planning a funeral or memorial, and the disposition of the body of yourself or a loved one. Knowledge of the Funeral Rule combined with an increased awareness of how the death merchants operate can provide you with your best protection as a consumer.

State Funeral and Cemetery Boards Tainted

The funeral directors and the cemetery operators boast of their stringent self-regulation which, if it were true, could give the consumer some comfort. In nearly every state, there are boards charged with the responsibility of overseeing the funeral and cemetery operations within those states. They are empowered to propose and adopt regulations to govern their respective industries.

These regulatory authorities are in most cases, little more than mouthpieces for the death merchants. In the makeup of the boards in most states, professionals from within the industries comprise the ruling majority, while consumer advocates are relegated to minority status (e.g., the state funeral board in Florida is comprised of five funeral directors—of whom no more than two can also have business connections with cemeteries—plus two consumers). Simply stated, these are committees of wolves watching the hen houses.

8

The Future of the Death Industry

Will the Funeral Business Adapt or Die?

"No matter who reigns, the merchant reigns."
Henry Ward Beecher, *Proverbs from Plymouth Pulpit* (1887)

The death merchants are always changing and fine-tuning the way they do business, seeking ways to adapt and grow at the same time. We've seen embalming become an American institution while the rest of the world regards it as an anomaly. We've seen burial vaults and liners, originally designed to thwart grave robbers, become "necessary" to keep out water and vermin and to prevent the ground from caving in. What changes are currently underway and what new ones might we expect to see in the future?

The Advent of the Giants

In recent years, the growth of conglomerates has cast a shadow over the single-owner funeral home and cemetery operations that for decades were fixtures on the American scene. Conglomerates presently own approximately 15% of all homes in the United States and more than one-fourth of all significant cemeteries are now owned by just three corporations.

Giant corporations are gobbling up the "mom and pop" funeral homes and cemeteries at a voracious rate. The largest, Service Corporation International (SCI), based in Houston, Texas, has more than 15,000 employees and posted annual revenues in 1995 of $1.5 billion. As of this writing, SCI owns 3,136 funeral homes and cemeteries worldwide—including more than 700 funeral homes and 175 cemeteries in the United States. In mid-1995, SCI purchased two of the largest funeral operations in Europe for $423 million, an acquisition that gave SCI about one-third of the funeral business in France plus sizable chunks in three other countries.

SCI chairman and chief executive officer, Robert L. Waltrip, said it's his goal to turn SCI into "the True Value Hardware of the funeral-service industry." Recognizing the value of local name recognition, however, SCI has slyly left the original names on the doors of the funeral homes it's acquired—no large True Value or Wal-Mart signs here. The public is largely unaware of the change in ownership. Why? Mr. Waltrip's protestations to the contrary, I believe the large conglomerates want to enjoy the rather massive discounts that are realized by buying goods and services in volume. At the same time, they relish the existing exorbitant mark-ups on those goods and services they inherited when they made their acquisitions. In other words, they want—and are getting—the "best" of both worlds.

The buying-power advantage of a conglomerate is obvious. But if a conglomerate has control of an entire segment of the market, will those savings be passed on to the consumer? That doesn't appear to be the case.

Funeral prices doubled in Dallas after a major conglomerate purchased several funeral homes there, according to an article in *Consumers Digest* (September/ October 1995). In its hometown of Houston, the corporation's funeral homes perform an average of 7,000 funerals per year (contrasted with just a few hundred handled by Houston's independent funeral homes). Houston has now become one of the most expensive places to die in the United States, the article quoted a prominent death-care advocate as saying.

The lucrative funeral home/cemetery acquisition business has an appetite that shows no signs of being satisfied.

Will the service that is the trademark of the locally owned funeral home be continued? Do most consumers want a multi-national conglomerate to handle their funerals? The answers are yet in the making, but I think that they would if properly done. When consumers buy such products as soft drinks and hamburgers, they most often do so on the basis of national reputation and name recognition. Despite the fact large corporations are slowly but steadily taking over, these conglomerates still believe at least some of the old ways of doing business are best. Therefore, they hang on to the small-town names and hide the presence of the real ownership.

I believe that if the death merchant conglomerates were to adopt the marketing and advertising philosophies of successful major chains in other industries, they would see a significant and positive impact in their business. People would recognize the buying power of the giants and would come to rely on receiving the same quality of service and selection of products coast to coast. Perhaps this will happen, but probably not for quite a while. For the time being, the giants are enjoying the fruits of their acquisitions without having to cut their over-inflated prices or to provide either continuity of service or management, all while assembling what portends to be a complete monopolization by these death merchants.

CASKET CLOSE-OUT SALE—Buy Today and Save!!

Ever wonder why you don't see a sale at a funeral home? Caskets and vaults are probably the only American consumer products that never go on sale, while every day you see sales for appliances, televisions, automobiles, etc.

When was the last time you were blasted by a radio or television commercial urging you to "Come on down and save today on caskets and vaults at Friendly Fred's Funeral Home"? Major retail chains have sales all the time, as do independent store owners. Why not funeral homes? Because they don't have to. They have secured for themselves a nearly competition-free marketplace and they have kept the consumers in the dark.

Independent funeral homes, however, are not taking the current corporate onslaught lying down. In one defensive maneuver, some independents are banding together to form purchasing cooperatives. They hope, of course, this move will enable them to enjoy at least some of the purchasing advantages of the bigger players. Other independents are merging with their own competitors in order to maintain market share and increase profitability. Following the example set by the larger conglomerates, however, any savings realized by these mini-conglomerates are counted as increased profits and not passed on to the consumers in the form of reduced prices.

Other independents are emphasizing the service aspect of their firms contrasted with that of the giant holding companies. Jean Wilson, vice president of Abbey Funeral Home in Tallahassee, Florida, is quoted in the *Funeral Service Insider* newsletter (August 14, 1995) as saying about service, "To be quite honest, the conglomerates are very easy to compete with. Going the extra mile is becoming a dinosaur."

Funerals with a Creative Flair

While the conglomerates are focusing on standardization of operations, controlling expenditures, streamlining management, and capitalizing on buying power, many independents are discovering a profitable niche through innovation. The entrepreneurial funeral director is freer to move and adapt to the changing market needs of the consumers.

For example, *The Wall Street Journal* (May 20, 1993) published an account of a funeral party (yes, a funeral party!) held in Sacramento, California: "In a hotel ballroom here, about 3,000 revelers float among bouquets of balloons and mingle around a trio of bars. An ice sculpture drips over the buffet. A seven-piece band, led by a vocalist in a black lace dress, blares out James Brown's 'I Feel Good.' In the midst of the action is the party's host—lying in a flag-draped coffin." The deceased, a California legislator and former Green Beret, had planned the party well in advance of his death and set aside the money to fund it.

Unconventional ceremonies may be an unexpected offshoot of the increasing numbers of pre-arranged funerals. People who are taking the time to "put their affairs in order" have more time to think about how they'd like their send-off to be.

A San Francisco bar owner, learning he had terminal cancer, arranged for a yacht cruise for 100 of his friends, according to *The Wall Street Journal* article. The cruise, for which the bar owner printed up invitations, was to take place the first Saturday after he died. Handing a friend the invitation, the bar owner said, "I'm having a party. I just don't have a date on it yet." The cruise took place, complete with a blues band, food and drink, and a scattering of the bar owner's ashes across the water.

Others have chosen to have their ashes packed in shells and fired from shotguns. Still others have them spread from airplanes and hot air balloons.

And why not? For those who enjoyed humor in life, why should they not plan on a little whimsy and celebration at the end? Granted, these avant-garde funerals are not likely to become standard funeral fare. Still, I believe, you will read more and more about these types of "celebrations of life" funerals in the future.

I understand that the drive-through viewing window at Junior Funeral Home in Pensacola, Florida, is no longer open (yes, it's true—you could drive up, take a gander at your pal, and sign the guest register, all without leaving the comfort of your car!). An increasing number of funeral establishments, however, are opening up businesses in strip malls across the country. So the return of the drive-through funeral home may be on the horizon.

Another shift, I believe, will be in the location of the funeral and memorial services. No, it does not have to be aboard a yacht or aloft in a hot air balloon, but I foresee an increasing number of services being held in places other than the traditional settings of the church, synagogue, and funeral home. More and more are being held in private homes, in parks, and even restaurants (usually in a private party room, however).

"Yet economics, along with political pressure, is a big incentive to change," wrote Jolie Solomon and Elizabeth Roberts in a *Newsweek* article (September 7, 1992). "Competition in the once courtly profession has forced some of the new tactics. Shifting customer fashions have forced others: embalming is out, cremation is in," they wrote. "For the mortician, whose biggest profits are in embalming, caskets and burial, the message is clear: adapt or die."

EERIE...BUT TRUE

Adapt or die has darkly humorous overtones to me. There have been many cases in which funeral directors had to cope with rival factions within a grieving family. Some "mourners" have come to funeral homes with guns in their pockets, aiming to disrupt the proceedings. We've even had fist fights break out during one of our viewings!

One of the most bizarre incidents, though, occurred when a young man murdered his mother. Not even a suspect at the time, the man came into the mortuary and calmly made the funeral arrangements. He subsequently attended the funeral and was apparently quite distraught over the loss. Shortly thereafter, he was arrested and confessed to committing the murder!

Interment on the Internet?

You've had your New Age funeral, now what do you do for an encore? Perhaps you'll consider being memorialized in cyberspace. The number of memorial sites on the World Wide Web is growing. Yes, you can place memorials—some with sound, some with pictures, and even some with videos—through your computer for virtually all the world to see. The cost of these memorials is relatively low, some charging a one-time $10 fee for text (with additional charges for graphics, sound, and video), while others are charging $10 and more per year.

I must admit, there is some appeal here. Visitors literally from around the world can stop by a memorial in one of these "cemeteries" and see biographical information about the deceased, view photographs and home videos, and listen to the deceased's favorite music. Several include hyperlinks—buttons—that the viewer can click on to jump to other Internet sites (e.g., a list of related e-mail addresses, areas of interest to the deceased, etc.). Some even allow visitors to leave "flowers" at the memorial.

These folks have even gotten on the pre-need bandwagon. At least one site offers the option of preplanning and prepaying your own cyber memorial. Why leave it to chance and Uncle Henry to write something about you? Better off doing it yourself!

If you're interested in visiting a virtual cemetery, you may want to drop in for a "stroll" through one of these:

The Cemetery Gate (http://www.funeral.net/info/ehtml/cemgate)—this one is run by the Armstrong Funeral Home, the same one we discussed in Chapter Two; **Cyber-Cemetery** (http://members.aol.com/

netgrave/); **Eternal Flame Commemorative Memorial Site** (http://www.eternalflame.com/); **Garden of Remembrance** (http://www.islandnet.com/~deathnet/gate.html); or **The World Wide Cemetery** (http://www.io.org/cemetery).

Cemeterians are beginning to embrace the idea of cemeteries in cyberspace. Some are considering offering to set up cyberplots as an added service to their consumers.

Thanatologists

The chameleon-like funeral directors (those folks once called "morticians" and "undertakers") and cemeterians (those people who used to run "graveyards") are slowly changing color once again in a move to gain yet another foothold in the death market. With increasing frequency, national and regional industry conventions include time on the agenda for *thanatologists*—experts in death.

This latest fad magically transforms funeral directors and cemeterians into "grief counselors," and it concerns me greatly. The training being offered is plainly profit-motivated. These folks have always postured themselves as sympathetic and empathetic individuals—even under their old titles. Hey, who knows? A handsomely framed certificate of training in grief counseling on the wall might just garner them a bit more respectability.

At the American Cemetery Association's (note: in 1996, the ACA changed its name to the International Cemetery and Funeral Association) 1995 convention and exposition held in Cincinnati, Ohio, members listened to an hour-long, emotional speech titled "The Funeral of the

Future: How Must Our Industry Serve a Changing Public?" The speaker urged the members to institute grief counseling programs at their cemeteries. Funeral directors are in touch with the families for only a few days following a death, while the actual grieving process is much longer, he said. Who in the death industry is in contact with families on a long-term basis? Why, the *cemetery operators*, he said supplying the answer to his own question. Better yet, he added, his research has shown that grief is a life-long process and, as such, could benefit from extremely long-term counseling (at a cost, no doubt).

I know from my own experience that grief is a personal and extended process. It varies widely, depending upon the individual. I also know, however, that if I needed professional guidance in interpreting and handling my grief, I would be more than just a little reluctant to attend a "grief seminar" held at a cemetery and led by someone who'd received a certificate of leadership following a five-day training seminar on the topic. While they may claim to be just the professional grief counselors you need, please remember that their sole purpose is to make themselves an integral part of your life to ensure your future patronage.

The funeral and cemetery businesses are just that— businesses. When you need a funeral, cremation, or burial plot, these are the people to see. When you need professional counseling to better understand and deal with any grief you might be experiencing, please seek an expert in the field.

'Til Death Do Us Part(?)

Funeral directors, always looking for a way to save a buck as well as make one, have begun to involve themselves in weddings. Weddings? Yes, weddings! A hearse is an expensive vehicle and much of the time just sits waiting in the garage until a new "passenger" calls. Let's get creative here. Some funeral homes are now renting their hearses and limousines for weddings, and other formal social events, and charging $125 per hour plus $75 per hour for the driver. I'm not certain how many takers they've had, just as I'm not certain just what image having a newly married couple depart in a hearse might make (for better or hearse perhaps?).

Now You See It, Now You Don't

Competition is a wonderful thing. There has been a recent influx of third-party casket sellers providing their goods directly to the consumers and at a considerable discount from the prices charged by funeral homes. Funeral directors have wasted no time countering this problem by appearing to discount their own caskets. When it comes to magically manipulating numbers, few can match the expertise of the death merchants.

To compete with the third-party casket sellers, some funeral homes are now only marking up the caskets they sell by 200%, instead of the 300% + that they used to. This is to make them appear more competitive. But hold on, they're not really about to give up the money, are they? No way. At the same time they are more fairly pricing their caskets, these funeral homes increase their basic services fee to accommodate the difference—plus probably make a few extra dollars.

In the August 28, 1995, issue of the *Funeral Service Insider* newsletter, an article quotes a funeral director as saying, "Recoup fifty percent of the profit you'd get on a traditional funeral by raising service charges $500-$700 and dropping casket costs $250-$500." Another funeral director, this one from Illinois, suggests increasing service charges three to four percent each year. He raises his charges, he said, quarterly (presumably whether they need to be increased or not!).

The Spying Game: How to Outfox Your Competition

I don't know whether or not the editors of the *Funeral Service Insider (FSI)* newsletter believe that no one but funeral directors will ever read their publication or whether they believe that all funeral directors must think alike. However, one of the more amazing articles I've ever read was contained in the August 14, 1995, issue of *FSI* and bore the title in the above subhead. The publication interviewed a "company spy" and offers the following suggestions:

• **One Man's Trash...**—A company trash barrel is "a rich trove of information." *FSI* does add the appropriate warning that plowing through dumpsters on private property is considered trespassing. As for shredded documents, the article said, "The more common strip shredding machines leave remains that can be reconstructed easily." What can the enterprising funeral sleuth expect to find in a competitor's garbage? Records of phone calls, supplier information, financial information, possible acquisition deals—to name just a few.

• **Competitor's Ex-Employees**—Interview these folks, it is suggested. "Disgruntled former employees can be a mother lode of information," the article says.

• **Amicable Departures**—Stay on good terms with your own employees who leave your funeral home, *FSI* offered. The thought is that these people might later be willing to reveal inside information about their new employers.

• **Check the Ads**—Classified advertisements, the article says, might tip you off to a competitor's defections and expansions. Another one of the hints is to read the competitor's hometown newspaper because, "You'll be surprised at what the competition will reveal to the locals."

• **Go Undercover**—Pretend to be an irate customer and call a competitor to learn how that funeral home treats its clients.

• **Salary Info**—Try and secure as much information as you can about the salaries being paid by competitors. Such data, the article says, can help "when you're faced with raiding competitors for top talent. Why pay more when you don't have to?"

I don't consider myself naïve. I am aware that corporate espionage occurs, but I don't condone it and I am astonished at seeing it being promoted so blatantly. I am reminded of an obituary I once read: "The talent of a meat-packer, the morals of a moneychanger and the manners of an undertaker."

Endless Supply of Customers

Fret not for the one-owner funeral home nor for the multi-national conglomerates. They will survive. They will continue to adapt. They will continue to organize into potent lobbying forces to protect their corporate turf. They will continue to manipulate the grief-stricken as they always have. Remember, though, for them to have customers, people must die.

Not to worry. The funeral and cemetery and crematory operators can always rely on a steady supply of customers. Death is their life (sorry, I couldn't resist!), and they track death statistics like a child devouring the baseball box scores in the morning newspaper. From 1950 to 1990, statistics show the death rate in the United States—as a percentage of total population—declined. But, because of the increase in the population during that time, the actual number of people dying is climbing each year. Nearly one percent of Americans die each year—that's at least 2.5 million customers right there.

The *Funeral Service Insider* newsletter regularly reports to its readers on the death rates throughout the major metropolitan areas in the United States. One such article (February 12, 1996) was headlined: "No pulse in 1995's fourth quarter death rate." Yes, I know it's morbid, but come on, put yourself in their shoes and try to get excited here. "The death rate was almost completely flat in 121 major cities in the United States during the fourth quarter of 1995 compared to 1994's fourth quarter...," the article reported. Bummer!

There was a ray of hope in the article in a section titled, "But look at this..." that revealed that the fourth quarter 1994 death rate wasn't as bad as the same quarter in 1993. Things might just be looking up. Maybe we're all going to keep dying after all. At last report, no cure for death was yet on the horizon. Was that a collective sigh of relief I just heard from those who get their profits from death?

9

The Ins and Outs of Prearranging

A Peek at the Pitfalls of Pre-Need Planning

"The buyer needs a hundred eyes, the seller not one."
George Herbert, *Jacula Prudentum* (1651)

The key to controlling future funeral and cemetery costs is to arrange and pay for them in advance. Unfortunately, this is easier said than done. There was, for a long time, much resistance to prearrangement contracts—particularly among the funeral directors.

Why? The answer is nothing more complicated than the fact that, in the funeral director's long experience, people will purchase more in an emotionally charged at-need moment than they will in a calmer and more stable pre-need moment. Cemeteries led the way in offering pre-need products, but now nearly all of the death merchants are being lured by the enormous sums of money available. Pre-need plans are being aggressively sold in the home, by phone, and through the mail.

Prearrangement Products: *Caveat Emptor*

Only about one-fourth of the population has made prearrangements and just slightly more than one-half of those have set aside any money to fund those prearrangements, according to the *1995 Study of American Attitudes Toward Ritualization and Memorialization*, prepared by The Wirthlin Group, of McLean, Virginia. Even so, more than $20 billion is already invested in various types of prearrangement contracts.

The majority of this money is in two types of basic products: trust funds and insurance policies. Sales of pre-need products (such things weren't even around just 20 or 30 years ago) will top four million contracts annually by the end of the century, by which time it's possible that more than half of all funerals will be prepaid. Most cemeteries, and more than half of all funeral homes, are now selling some type of pre-need plan. Others are also getting into the act. For example, our friend, Hillenbrand Industries (remember the manufacturer of Batesville Caskets and American Tourister luggage we discussed in Chapter Two?), also owns Forethought Life. In business for just 10 years, this company has sold nearly $2 billion in pre-need products through 4,000 funeral homes located in 41 states.

Sadly, there is little being done to monitor these funds or the people in charge of them. At the present time, there are no federal laws regulating pre-need products. As a result, more and more stories are surfacing in which pre-need monies are being mishandled and, in some cases, stolen. The victims are often the elderly (they're targeted by pre-need marketers since more than 70% of deaths occur among persons 65 or older and, thus, are more likely considering making prearrangements) who are unable to shrug off such a financial loss.

As discussed earlier, the FTC is responsible for enforcing the Funeral Rule, but that admittedly limited regulation addresses only funeral expenses and does not cover the sales of most pre-need products. While its purview encompasses deceptive trade practices, the FTC has not taken it upon itself to actively pursue the matter of pre-need fraud.

Felt pressured into signing your pre-need contract? Consumers should be aware of the FTC's "Cooling-Off" Rule that gives buyers three business days to cancel a contract signed in the consumer's home or otherwise away from the seller's place of business.

In 1995, seven pre-need carriers (American Funeral Assurance Company, Brookings International Life Insurance Company, Forethought Life, Homesteaders Life, Pan-Western Life, Pierce National Life, and United Family Life) petitioned the FTC, asking the agency to waive the Cooling-Off Rule contending they were already regulated by the FTC's Funeral Rule. The petitioners claimed the high-pressure sales tactics for which the rule was intended did not occur in pre-need sales presentations. In the spring of 1996, the FTC ruled that the Cooling-Off Rule must apply, stating that the Funeral Rule doesn't provide consumers with information regarding canceling a pre-need contract. As perhaps a gentle jab, the FTC added that there is nothing preventing sellers from providing a cancellation right that exceeds the three days and suggested a 30-day period would be perfectly acceptable.

Moving to fill the federal legislative vacuum, some states have taken it upon themselves to address the matter, but their efforts have resulted in a maze of confusing, conflicting, and often inadequate laws. Many states have one set of regulations governing funeral homes and another for cemeteries.

SOME SILLY STATE STATUTES

• Some states (e.g., New York and New Jersey) stipulate that funeral merchandise can only be sold by funeral directors and by no one else.

• Some states (e.g., Tennessee) only allow funeral directors to sell vaults.

• Some states (e.g., Michigan, New York, and Wisconsin) do not allow funeral homes and cemeteries to be owned by the same people.

• Some states (e.g., Ohio) require cemeteries to be not-for-profit organizations, partnerships, or proprietorships.

• Some states (e.g., South Carolina) do not allow the sale of insurance as a pre-need vehicle.

• Some states require that a funeral director be present at a funeral or a viewing.

Thanks to the powerful lobbying efforts of the death merchants, these and other laws have been enacted with the end result of reducing competition and inflating prices.

Only three states (i.e., Arizona, Iowa, and Louisiana) annually conduct on-site audits of pre-need books, while the other states and the District of Columbia either require only an annual report be submitted and conduct on-site checks every three or four years.

Who's in charge? In some states, the responsibility for inspection rests with the banking commissions, while in others it's vested in the state funeral/cemetery boards (which, as you will recall, are merely extensions of the industry as the majority of members are professionals from within the business). In the states where there are neither boards nor agencies specifically assigned to oversee the pre-need funds, the task usually falls to the attorneys general.

However, please don't be dissuaded from prearranging! I cannot overemphasize how important it is for everyone to do as much preplanning and prepaying of their funeral and cemetery needs as possible. This is the best way in which the consumer can reduce the high cost of dying (in my own experience, I found that most people will spend about a third less when making prearrangements than at a time of need) and avoid the stress of making the arrangements on an at-need basis. Also, it has the additional advantage of helping make certain that you will get the type of funeral and disposition you want.

What You Are Prearranging

A cemetery pre-need package often consists of a couple of plots, a bronze memorial, a pair of vaults or mausoleum crypts, and perhaps the opening and closing of the graves or crypts. The process is fairly simple. You sign a contract and the cemetery gives you a deed for the plots and a certificate of ownership for the merchandise you purchased. The deed for the plots is not a deed for the property itself, but rather a deed for the interment rights in those plots (you only have the right to inter dead human remains in the property; you can't open a small coffee shop or build a tiny get-away cabin).

EERIE...BUT TRUE...*and* INTERESTING

An anomaly of the pre-need purchases made through cemeteries, however, is that the consumer may be asked to pay interest on the goods for the entire life of the contract.

We have become accustomed, of course, to paying interest charges on nearly all the installment-payment purchases we make (e.g., refrigerators, cars, televisions, etc.). The difference is that when we buy refrigerators, cars, and televisions, we take them home and use them. The consumer may not have need for—and, therefore, won't take delivery on—the cemetery plot, vault, and memorial for decades after they were purchased. Charging it is perfectly legal but avoidable by the consumer. I have never heard of a funeral home charging interest on any pre-need purchase. The consumer can find the same or comparable vaults and memorials at a funeral home and not have to pay a penny in interest.

A funeral pre-need package is normally comprised of a casket or some type of container, plus whatever services are selected (e.g., embalming, cremation, visitation, transportation, memorial service, etc.). The funeral package may, in some instances, also include a vault and memorial.

Trust Funds

Between 30% and 70% of the money you invest in a cemetery prearrangement contract—it varies according to the laws of the particular state—is required to be set aside in a trust fund to cover the price of the merchandise purchased. Funeral plans, on the other hand, are often required to trust much higher amounts, sometimes as high as 100%.

The difference in trusting percentages between the funeral and cemetery industries is reflective of the dichotomy of their respective business philosophies. Funeral homes prefer the higher trusting amount as it virtually locks the consumer in and it inhibits competition (from a competitor's standpoint, it's extremely difficult and expensive to sell against an investment in which nearly all of the customer's money is placed in trust, especially when you also have to fund advertising and high commission payouts to sales representatives).

On the surface, 100% trusting appears to be a strong argument on behalf of the consumer. Even with all of the money trusted, however, these plans do not guarantee the consumer that the funds invested will actually cover the cost of the funeral. The reason is that the funeral plans are predicated on retail prices, whereas the cemetery plans are based on wholesale prices. If the plan is based on wholesale prices, less needs to be trusted to ensure future coverage of expenses than if the plan is based on retail prices.

Even just a third of the money trusted (provided, of course, it is prudently invested) is widely regarded as sufficient to guarantee that the goods (e.g., a vault) can be purchased at wholesale whenever in the future the death occurs. Funeral homes, however, will sell the same vault, place 100% of the funds in trust, and still not guarantee the price. If the merchandise retails for more than what the trust account earns, the difference will be charged to the consumer (conversely, the consumer should get a dollar-for-dollar refund if the actual purchase price is less than the amount of the funds in trust).

The amount of the investment not placed in trust is available to the death merchants to use entirely at their discretion. Also, when the monies in trust grow through interest to a point where they are greater than the amount needed to purchase the selected merchandise as determined at the time the contract is written, the excess dollars can often be taken out of the trust as profit to the seller.

Of course, the argument should not be what the funeral homes and cemeteries want, but rather what is in the best interest of the consumer. My personal opinion is that all of the trusted money should remain trusted for the protection of the consumer. What if the trust were, in the future, to experience a financial reversal and decrease in overall value to the point where the funds were no longer sufficient to cover the cost of the merchandise? Who would pay the difference? Presumably, the cemetery or funeral home would be liable for the shortfall. But what if the reversals were so large as to force the company into bankruptcy?

I found it interesting that in several of my meetings with representatives of the American Association of

Retired Persons (AARP)—a strong lobby in its own right—they frequently endorsed the funeral directors' approach to trusting. The funeral folks apparently convinced the AARP that the consumer is better protected by the higher percentage of funds trusted. The AARP apparently gave little consideration to the fact that pre-need plans need to provide assurance that the cost of the eventual funeral will be covered. To its credit, however, the AARP recently hired a researcher to review the pre-need laws of all 50 states.

Portability

As long as the consumer uses the cemetery or funeral home where the pre-need contract was written, there should be no problem. However, if the consumer moves, the pre-need contract may not be transferable. The new company most likely will charge the consumer the current prices for the same goods and services, and will only credit the consumer with the amount already paid into the trust fund.

Funeral homes will not honor pre-need contracts purchased at another facility because they claim prices and products and services are so different that there is no way they can supply anything similar. The consumer who wants to transfer a pre-need program is left with few options and often ends up paying an additional 50% to 100% beyond what's already been invested. Pardon me, but that's utter nonsense—we're only talking about widely available caskets and vaults and basic funeral services here. There is no reason why they cannot, and should not, accommodate the consumer (they will gain the good will of a satisfied customer and likely increased business through the customer's family and friends).

ARE YOU SURE YOU *CAN* TAKE IT WITH YOU?

Portability should be one of the primary concerns when purchasing death merchandise and services on a pre-need basis. Take, for example, a consumer who selects a bronze memorial retailing for $1,000 at Cemetery "A" and pays $1,000 into a prearrangement contract with that cemetery. The consumer is guaranteed to receive the memorial, paid in full, from the cemetery, at the time of death. Cemetery "A" trusts 40% of the amount—or $400—sufficient to enable the cemetery to deliver the memorial when needed.

Our consumer, however, relocates and contacts Cemetery "B" in the new town. There, the consumer learns that the same memorial now retails for $2,000 and, upon transferring the prearrangement contract, is told another $1,000 must be paid before the memorial will be delivered.

One possible solution would be to request that Cemetery "A" deliver the original memorial to the consumer and refund the amount charged for installation. This way, the consumer could personally take the memorial to Cemetery "B" and simply pay the new cemetery's installation charge.

From the cemeteries' standpoint, there are two obvious solutions, were they to be cooperative: (1) Cemetery "A" could ship the memorial to the new cemetery; and (2) Cemetery "A" could transfer the trusted monies to Cemetery "B" so that the new cemetery could purchase the memorial when it was needed by the consumer. As for the grave plots themselves, and the opening and closing charges, the new cemetery should be happy to either accept the deed for the lots (remember, the cost to the cemetery is only about $25 per plot) and, in the transaction, receive a new customer and probably referrals.

Instead, most cemeteries continue to penalize consumers who want to transfer their pre-need investments. Even the International Cemetery and Funeral Association's highly touted—mostly by the ICFA itself—"cemetery exchange" program, supposedly the model of portability, operates this way. Perhaps the ICFA is concerned about potential liability for sanctioning the penalties described above, as it has established a separate non-profit corporation to handle the portability issue.

It's no wonder consumers are going to need grief therapy.

Consumers should insist on complete portability— complete item-for-item exchange as opposed to a dollar-for-dollar exchange. Consumers should not buy any pre-need goods and services unless guaranteed in writing that they have the right to take those same goods and services to any other facility in the country. If the goods cannot be shipped, then the consumer should at least be able to buy the same goods—at the original price and using the funds already invested—at the new location. Also, there should be no penalty to the consumer (some states permit penalties of loss of interest and some include a percentage of the principal when transferring pre-need plans). Simply stated: item-for-item portability is good; dollar-for-dollar is bad.

What's a Consumer to Do?

Consumers can place the money in trust themselves and avoid the funeral director and the cemetery operator altogether. In fact, many people do just that. The major advantage is that the individual is in control of how and where the money is invested. The major disadvantages to this approach, though, are that it leaves the money in the estate and exposed to taxation, and if there are too many assets in the estate, there may be potential problems qualifying for Medicare and Medicaid benefits.

A slightly better approach, if it's available in your community, is to find a funeral home or cemetery that has an established trust account at a local financial institution that provides the trusteeship of the monies. As trustee, the financial institution will be entitled to collect some fees, but that would be a reasonable trade-off for receiving good stewardship of the funds. Be wary of prearrangement contracts in which an independent individual or individuals—*particularly* the funeral director or cemetery operator—oversee the monies in the trust fund. This is the riskiest way for consumers to have their money invested. There have been instances in which such funds were placed in rare coins and other similarly volatile investments, the monies lost, and the investors left with no meaningful recourse.

Some states have organized master trust associations in which many funeral homes participate. The ones of which I'm aware are managed in an extremely conservative manner and have not realized the returns of the more progressive funds. Not a bad approach, though, as long as the funds keep pace with inflation. There are some negatives, of course. If the amount in an individual's trust fund is insufficient to pay for the goods and services ordered, the family will be forced to pay the balance. Two other negatives to the master trust funds are the cost to the consumer of having to pay someone to manage the money, and that frequently the association receives some type of kick-back fee ranging from .25% to .5% of the monies invested.

Revocable vs. Irrevocable

Consumers, even those dependent upon Social Security and who qualify for Medicare and Medicaid, can establish an irrevocable (i.e., the money cannot be removed) trust, bank account, or insurance policy— provided the funds are used exclusively for funeral and cemetery expenses. An alternative for these folks is to set up a revocable trust (i.e., the money can be removed). You can't, however, have both.

Questions You Should Ask about Pre-Need Trusts

If you choose to fund your future death expenses through a trust, these are some questions you should ask before proceeding:

1. Who is the trustee of the fund? (It is a conflict of interest for someone in the funeral home or cemetery to be the trustee, although this is allowed in some states—due primarily to strong industry lobbying.)

2. Who sets up the trust (is it the funeral home, cemetery, or an outside person)?

3. How much are the trustee fees? (.7% to 1.25% maximum—the higher the amount trusted, the lower the fee; larger trustee fees often indicate that there are kick-backs being paid to the funeral home, cemetery operator, industry association, or someone.)

4. What investments have been made by the trust? (Ask for a listing of the investments. If the trust is invested in mutual funds, be aware these funds might charge their own fee of 2% to 5% plus another 1% to 2% annually. If the trust is invested in high-fee mutual funds, I suggest running in the opposite direction as fast as you can!)

5. What are the historic returns on the trust monies invested?

6. Is the trust truly portable? (It should be a plan recognized and accepted throughout the United States whereby the monies can be used item-for-item—and without penalty—by any other funeral and/or cemetery facility you choose.)

7. What state agency, if any, oversees the trust fund? (Then ask that agency for a report on the trust fund. You will learn a lot about the fund, and it will show you when the fund was last audited.)

8. Can the funeral arrangements you make be changed by family members and, if so, what can you do prevent that from happening?

9. Is this an individual trust fund? (It shouldn't be unless required by law. The fees will probably be higher—so, again, avoid this type at all costs.)

10. Is it a revocable or irrevocable trust? (In other words, can you get your money back?)

11. Is it federally insured? (Take advantage of this whenever possible.)

Insurance Policies Are Best

The other major method for funding pre-need, particularly funerals, is through some type of insurance (insurance policies are the basis of most pre-need programs sold by funeral directors). In my opinion, insurance policies are the best way to go. The insurance industry is highly regulated. Also, insurance companies are typically more balanced and more stable than most death merchants. Even when insurance companies go bankrupt, state and federal agencies often come to the rescue of the policyholders. Certainly the same cannot be said of funeral homes and cemeteries!

There are three basic types of policies:

Dollar-For-Dollar Coverage—in which the customer pays, for example, $4,000 in premiums for a policy with a face value of $4,000. Assuming that today's funeral might cost $4,000, about the only positive with this type is that the customer is making some pre-need arrangements. The negatives are that the customer has grossly overpaid for the policy and still has no guarantee that the face value of the policy will cover the cost of the funeral when it eventually occurs. By all means, avoid purchasing this type of coverage.

Today's Dollars for Tomorrow's Funeral Costs—in which the customer pays approximately $4,000 in premiums for a policy with a face value of $6,000 to $8,000. In addition to making pre-need arrangements, the only other positive is that the customer's estate will get money back if the cost of the funeral is less than that of the policy's face amount. The negatives still outweigh the positives. The consumer has again overpaid for the policy and there is no guarantee that the policy will cover the eventual costs of the funeral. A better deal, obviously, than the first example, but still not a very good bargain.

Insurance That Grows in Value—in which the customer pays approximately $2,500 in premiums for a policy with a face amount of $4,000 (for this example, the estimated cost of a funeral today) is the best possible type of coverage. This type of policy is designed to increase in face value at roughly the rate of inflation. The consumer has made pre-need arrangements and received the most value for the dollars invested. Assuming the insurance company is financially sound and the funeral director guarantees that the policy will cover the cost of the funeral no matter when it occurs, there really are no negatives to this type of coverage.

Questions You Should Ask about Pre-Need Insurance Policies

Even though insurance is your best bet, there are still some things you will want to know before buying a policy:

1. What are the premiums vs. the face value of the policy?

2. Is the policy guaranteed to cover the cost of the merchandise and services you've selected? (Do not accept the policy if it is not *guaranteed* by the funeral director to cover the cost.)

3. What is the growth potential of the policy?

4. What is the rating of the insurance company?

5. What state agency oversees insurance sales in your state? (Contact that agency and request information on the company.)

6. What commission is being paid? (The seller has to answer!)

7. Who is the beneficiary? (It should be the funeral home, and not your estate if you want to avoid taxation. But, again, the funeral home must guarantee that the policy will cover the funeral and goods selected.)

Just How Final *Are* Your Final Arrangements?

So, you've made your prearrangement plans and arranged to pay for those plans. Everything's set in stone. Right? *Wrong.* The death merchants, it seems, have their own chisel. They are ready for you—or rather your survivors—on this one. Since people who preplan funerals frequently spend far less than they would at the time of death, funeral directors have devised a strategy to increase the cost of your funeral *after* your death. They will do this by manipulating your emotionally distraught family members into changing your plans and spending more money. As repugnant as this thought is, it is happening. At this time, only two states—Texas and Washington—have enacted laws that protect the wishes of the deceased.

Paul Irion, the religious affairs coordinator for the National Funeral Directors Association, wrote in the NFDA's magazine, *The Director* (March 1996): "We have to be aware, however, of some possible limitations in prearrangement which require that we pay special attention to the needs of families when death occurs. It would be so easy to take prearrangement literally and to assume that nothing remains to be done when the time of need arrives."

What does he mean it "would be so easy to take prearrangement literally?" Of course, it's easy—it's also the ethical and moral responsibility of the family *and* the death merchants to take the prearrangement plans literally!

"Funeral directors and participating clergy," Irion continues, "should review in detail all of the prearrangement plans with family members. Because these plans were made without knowing what the particular needs of the family would be at the time of death, mourners should be asked, 'Are you comfortable with these plans?' If not, discuss ways in which those needs could be met." He offers, as an example, a prearrangement plan which stipulated immediate disposition of the body. Perhaps, he suggests, the family would rather have "wanted the kind of support that comes from friends through a funeral."

The primary purpose behind the thoughtfulness of prearranging is to protect surviving loved ones from having to go through this type of coercion on the worst day of their lives. How dare these supposedly caring and sensitive death professionals defy the wishes of the deceased and prey on the surviving members of the family! And to involve their friends, the clergy?

Irion adds, "It is a great advantage to talk to the clergy with whom you work about this concern for the possible loss of family involvement when a prearrangement is being carried out. Clergy need to understand their special responsibility to involve the family, supporting the reality of their loss. Talk with your clergy colleagues about ways in which families can be helped to express their sense of loss when they have little part in the actual arranging of the funeral."

He concludes by acknowledging that prearrangement can be "a very good thing," but adds, "...we need to know that serving a family well means that we find ways to involve them actively in the funeral process, so that they benefit from the therapeutic value of that experience." Spare me, Mr. Irion...please.

Bruce Overton, NFDA president, says in a separate article in that same issue of *The Director*, "The truth is that preneed makes a lot of sense for many but not for all. It may be in our rush to preplan, we are denying families the very positive and healing exercise of making funeral arrangements for someone dear to them." He added, "Survivors should be permitted to regain their status in memorialization planning."

Once you're deceased you can't very well reach out and grab the funeral director by his nice black lapels, shake him, and yell, "This is what I wanted and this is the way it *will* be!" Your only alternative is to involve all family members in the preplanning process. Let them know how important it is to you that the arrangements be carried out as you have planned. Warn them of the piranha disguised as the caring undertaker who will pounce on them once you've passed away.

Be Wary—But Be a Buyer

I know there are a lot of pitfalls to buying your funeral and cemetery goods and services on a pre-need basis, but the positives far outweigh the negatives. Preplanning is absolutely the best thing you can do to ensure that you get the final arrangements you want and save money at the same time.

I recommend you preplan your needs and arrange to pay for them through an insurance policy guaranteed to cover those cost of those needs. By properly preplanning and prepaying, you can lock in today's prices and save up to 50% over what you or your survivors will be forced to pay if you choose to do nothing.

10

Getting the Funeral You Want

A Guide to Purchasing

"The time to repair the roof is when the sun is shining."
John F. Kennedy, *State of the Union Message* (1962)

Well, my friends, we've covered a lot of territory. Now I'd like to share some thoughts on ways you can get the funeral or cremation you desire for the price you are willing to pay. Hopefully, the information contained so far has done much to prepare you as a consumer.

How Much Should It Cost?

The prices charged by the death merchants continue to rise year after year. In March 1996, the average funeral, including the casket, cost $4,281—that's up 3.5% from the previous year (by contrast, the average cost 10 years ago was just $2,516). The price of the average outer burial rose to $781 in 1996—up more than 3% in just one year. The costs of cremations, cemetery charges, and the prices of all other goods and services are also on the increase.

By the time you add together *all* the average funeral and cemetery charges, the final bill frequently runs between $7,000 and $8,000. Obviously, you can spend more if you prefer (and wouldn't the funeral directors and cemetery operators be happy little campers if you did?).

Can you spend less? Absolutely. Here is a list of ways to dispose of a body, from the least expensive to the most expensive, using 1996 prices (not included is the cost of picking up the body, delivering it to the funeral home, crematorium, and/or cemetery—this cost will normally vary according to the distance traveled):

Donation of Body—A body donated to a medical school will be cremated when the school is finished with it and, if desired, the cremains will be returned to the family. While homeless persons, without any known family members, provide the majority of donated bodies, it is becoming more fashionable and acceptable for others as well. By donating your body, you will have aided in the education of future medical personnel, helped in the research against disease, and your family will have received the cremation—all at little or no cost (some expenses for transporting the body may be incurred). A sample body donation form is included [Appendix VI]. You should be aware, though, that a considerable amount of time may elapse between the time the body is donated and when you receive the cremains. TOTAL AVERAGE COST: $0-$200.

Direct Cremation—One of the least expensive ways of disposing of a body is to not have it embalmed and send it directly to cremation in a low-cost container (you can save even more if you're comfortable using no container at all) and without purchasing any other goods and services. The price is governed primarily by the amount of competition for cremation business in the area.

The ashes will be placed in a cardboard box or plastic container and given to the family for disposition, frequently for scattering. TOTAL AVERAGE COST: $400-$700.

Other Optional Cremation Expenses: If you prefer, you can purchase a simple urn for approximately $150, or more elaborate ones for as much as $2,000 and more. You can count on spending an additional several hundred dollars to several thousands of dollars if you opt for placing the cremains in a burial site, columbaria, or mausoleum. These additional choices can escalate the total cost of cremation to rival that of a traditional funeral and burial.

Direct Burial—An unembalmed body buried in the least expensive casket without a viewing or a funeral (other than a graveside service) will cost somewhat more than a direct cremation. The bill for a direct burial should include these approximate amounts: $500 for the casket, $250 for the cemetery lot, $350 for the cost of opening and closing the grave, $200 for a basic concrete grave liner, and $500 for a small flat marker for the grave. TOTAL AVERAGE COST: $1,800.

Cremation with Memorial Service—To the cost of a direct cremation, add the cost of the memorial service at a funeral home or crematory ($300) and the rental of a modest casket ($700). TOTAL AVERAGE COST: $1,400-$1,700.

Traditional Funeral and In-Ground Burial—Add the cost of embalming (average = $400) and the cost of the funeral at the mortuary (average = $800 to $1,200) to the cost for a Direct Burial. TOTAL AVERAGE COST: $3,000-$3,400.

Traditional Funeral and Immurement in a Mausoleum—The costs of mausoleum crypts can vary widely, depending upon size and construction, and can be as high as $15,000 or more (average = $1,000 to $2,500). Add in the cost of the casket (average = $500), the crypt marker (average = $500), and the cost of the funeral service (average = $800 to $1,200). TOTAL AVERAGE COST: $2,800-$4,700.

Getting the funeral and disposition you want for the price you're willing to pay will take some work on your part. Apart from perhaps buying a home and a car, this will probably be one of the most expensive purchases you will make during your lifetime. Here are some ways you can save on costs without sacrificing quality:

Ten Tips for Saving Money

1. **Prearranging**—Avoid making important personal and financial decisions under the emotional duress when a death occurs. Prearrange and prepay for the funeral and the disposition of the body.

2. **Considering Cremation**—The act of cremation may run counter to your religious or secular beliefs. If not, then cremation may be the most economical choice you can make. Just make certain that you make the choices with which *you* are comfortable. As for the cremains, the scattering of ashes is enjoying a resurgence of popularity and the process can be an emotionally cathartic one. If this is not your choice, your options are to place them in a grave or columbaria at additional cost, or to keep the cremains at home in an urn.

3. **Selecting the Funeral Home**—Please take the time to shop around. The FTC's Funeral Rule is there to assist you. Use it to your advantage. Let your fingers do the walking at first and call several funeral homes and ask their prices—they're required to give them to you over the phone, but only if you ask! Narrow the selection down to at least two or three and then make personal visits. If your family or friends have used them before and were satisfied with the service and the price, let this information be but *part* of your decision-making process. Trust your instincts. Did you get the information you requested? Did you feel as though the funeral director and staff had your best interests at heart, or did you sense that the profit motive was at work during your meeting? Be wary of disclosing personal financial information. Were your requests taken seriously, or did you perceive an attempt to steer you in a different direction? Most importantly, take the written price lists home and compare before making a decision. Avoid the temptation and the pressure to be done with it by signing a contract right there on the spot.

4. **Casket Selection**—Explore your options here, as well. Thanks to the FTC's Funeral Rule, a whole new industry is emerging. Third-party casket sellers will no doubt offer you the best deal. The funeral home is required to assist you in your funeral arrangements even if you purchase your casket from another source, and it is illegal for them to tack on a surcharge or handling fee if you do. In selecting the casket, bear in mind that its primary purpose is for show. When you think about it, the casket is actually seen for only about six to eight hours, even in a traditional service. After that, it goes into the ground to disintegrate.

Your own personal needs must guide you here. As for sealer versus non-sealer caskets, I urge you to resist the temptation to pay additional money for a sealing casket, believing it will provide significant additional protection—it won't.

5. **Vault Selection**—Much of what applies to casket selection also applies to selecting the vault. Check out third-party vendors (they may not be permitted, depending upon the lobbying abilities of your particular state's funeral and cemetery boards). First, of course, make certain that the cemetery you've selected actually requires a grave vault or liner (they probably do). I recommend you select the least expensive grave liner possible, avoiding the more expensive vaults (especially those with gaskets, epoxy, or other special sealers).

6. **Selecting a Grave Marker**—The most economical grave markers will probably be found at local monument dealers and the most expensive at cemeteries. If you follow this tip and purchase the memorial from a third-party vendor, be sure and check with the cemetery first to determine what restrictions they place on the type and size of marker. Also, ask what cemetery labor charges you'll have to pay to have the marker installed. Ask what restrictions they would place on you were you to have the marker installed yourself.

7. **Opening/Closing the Grave**—If you can find an excavation company that will handle these chores for you and that can satisfy whatever legal and financial roadblocks the cemetery will attempt to place in its way,

I believe you can realize savings of up to 50% over what the cemetery will charge you.

8. **Choosing the Location for the Service**—The funeral home is the probably the most expensive site you could pick to hold the funeral service. Your other options are many, and I encourage you to explore them. Although the funeral home will charge you to transport the body to another location for the service, you will still save a great deal of money. Your church or temple is no doubt the least expensive and, in most cases, there is no charge. Some fraternal and veterans organizations have their own lodges and meeting halls. These are frequently made available for funeral services for their members and the cost, if any, is usually quite minimal. There is also the possibility of a wake, traditionally a gathering of family and friends before the body is buried. I personally believe wakes are more emotionally restorative to the survivors than the normally more staid and somber viewings. Before the development of the modern funeral home, the wakes were usually held in the family's home with the body present. While you probably don't want to have the body delivered to your house, I still encourage you to consider having an old-fashioned wake there (the cost is minimal, friends routinely will bring food and drink, and the results might prove emotionally healthy). Beyond these ideas, let your imagination be your guide.

9. **Exploring Vehicle Options**—Only one funeral home vehicle is normally required. Unless you want to place the casket in the back of your four-wheel-drive truck, you will probably want to utilize the hearse. To save money, use private cars and avoid the cost of limousines for the

family, clergy, and pallbearers, and the cost of another funeral home vehicle for the flowers. Friends would no doubt be honored and readily willing to accept were you to ask them to serve as drivers.

10. **Eliminating the Frills**—Avoid the temptation of one-stop shopping at the funeral home. Guest registers, thank you and remembrance cards, prayer cards, etc., are not expensive items; but they do add up, especially when the funeral home's mark-up is factored in. Also, be certain that you've contacted all friends, family, and associates who could serve as pallbearers before hiring the funeral home's professional staff to carry the casket. All of these—the incidental items and the pallbearers—if handled by the family and friends, can actually serve as a valuable part of the grieving/healing process.

Conclusion

I want to reiterate that many of the people I met during my years in the business were fine, upstanding people. As with any industry, there are malcontents, misfits, and miscreants. By and large, they are good folks, but they are business people first and foremost. Their motives are too often fueled by profit and misguided by greed.

How can they justify their actions? You need to understand that funeral directors and cemetery owners believe in their heart of hearts that you do not want or need to have the kind of information presented in this book. They do this by making several assumptions:

• They *assume* you are simply not interested in the knowledge. They believe that you are best served by them selling you what you want. But, at the same time, they are not willing to share with you the information you need with which to make informed decisions.

• They *assume* you want to have the body of the deceased protected from the elements and, therefore, purposely perpetuate the myth of protection as they try to sell you sealing caskets and vaults.

• They *assume* you want to buy your way into the heart of a loved one by spending as much as you can possibly afford (and perhaps more).

• They *assume* you are actually going to feel better and deal more easily with your grief if you buy the most expensive casket and services and the most expensive burial plot.

• They *assume* you want to purchase the best for the most in order to show families and friends just how much you cared for the deceased.

These assumptions—myths, if you will—have been perpetuated for generations by the death merchants. The vast majority of funeral directors and cemetery operators subscribe to them without question.

Also, let's remember that funeral directors and cemetery owners find themselves in a contradictory position. Most of these people purport that they want to do what is right by the families and to serve them in the best possible way. That benevolent spirit, however, often conflicts with their business responsibilities to increase their sales and maximize profits.

This conflict makes it easy to understand why death merchants opt for the choice that will render the greatest profitability to themselves and their operations. This is not, in itself, necessarily wrong. It is, in fact, what every successful business operator must do—sell the most products at the highest prices for the greatest profits possible.

There is one glaring difference, however, between the industries of the death merchants and all other types of businesses. There is much more consumer knowledge available about nearly every type of business operation *other* than that of the death merchants. Consumers seldom allow themselves to be taken advantage of when buying a car, for example. They can get information about the average wholesale/retail price of the car, know what their bargaining position will be before they walk into the dealership, and shop around in order to get the most features for the best price. When it comes to purchasing funeral and cemetery goods and services, however, the consumer woefully lacks the basic knowledge about what choices are available and what they should cost.

My sincere hope is that I have helped increase your knowledge and understanding of the funeral, cemetery, and allied businesses, and that this book will assist you in making wiser, more informed decisions.

About the Author

Until his retirement in the fall of 1994, Darryl J. Roberts spent his entire life in and around the funeral and cemetery industries. Born on November 12, 1944, he was already helping with his father's cemetery business in Beckley, West Virginia, by the age of twelve.

Mr. Roberts received his B.S. Degree in Business from the University of Tennessee in 1967, and continued with post-graduate studies at the West Virginia College of Graduate Studies. He is married and has one son.

In the summers during college, he began his professional career as a memorial counselor selling cemetery lots. After graduation, he became manager of one of his father's corporate properties in Richlands, Virginia. Upon his father's death in 1980, Mr. Roberts was named president of the corporation which consisted of 26 cemeteries and three funeral homes. While president, he produced the award-winning sales video titled *Till Death Do Us Part*, the first professionally produced sales training video in the industry. He was chief executive officer of the company until 1994.

He served on the board of directors of the West Virginia Cemetery Association from 1970 to 1978, served as its president from 1974 to 1975, and was elected president emeritus of the association in 1993. He was also a member of the board of directors of the Pre-Arrangement Association of America from 1972 to 1980, and served as its president from 1975 to 1976. In addition, he served on the board of directors of the Ohio Association of Cemeteries from 1976 to 1978. He was a founding member of the Cemetery Service Council—an organization designed to assist consumers and cemeteries in the resolution of disputes—and served as its president in 1983. Over the years, Mr. Roberts was a featured speaker at numerous state, regional, and national meetings of the funeral and cemetery industries.

Appendix I

Funeral Rule

Part 453—Funeral Industry Practices Revised Rule

Section:
453.1 Definitions
453.2 Price Disclosures
453.3 Misrepresentation
453.4 Required Purchase of Funeral Goods or Funeral Services
453.5 Services Provided without Prior Approval
453.6 Retention of Documents
453.7 Comprehension of Disclosures
453.8 Declaration of Intent
453.9 State Exemptions

Authority: 15 U.S.C. 57a(a); 15 U.S.C. 46(g); 5 U.S.C. 552

453.1 Definitions
   (a) <u>Alternative Container</u> An "alternative container" is an unfinished wood box or other non-metal receptacle or enclosure, without ornamentation or a fixed interior lining, which is designed for the encasement of human remains and which is made of fiberboard, pressed-wood, composition materials (with or without an outside covering) or like materials.

(b) <u>Cash Advance Item</u> A "cash advance item" is any item of service or merchandise described to a purchaser as a "cash advance," "accommodation," "cash disbursement," or similar term. A cash advance item is also any item obtained from a third party and paid for by the funeral provider on the purchaser's behalf. Cash advance items may include, but are not limited to: cemetery or crematory services; pallbearers; public transportation; clergy honoraria; flowers; musicians or singers; nurses; obituary notices; gratuities; and death certificates.

(c) <u>Casket</u> A "casket" is a rigid container which is designed for the encasement of human remains and which is usually constructed of wood, metal, fiberglass, plastic, or like material, and ornamented and lined with fabric.

(d) <u>Commission</u> "Commission" refers to the Federal Trade Commission.

(e) <u>Cremation</u> "Cremation" is a heating process which incinerates human remains.

(f) <u>Crematory</u> A "crematory" is any person, partnership, or corporation that performs cremation and sells funeral goods.

(g) <u>Direct Cremation</u> A "direct cremation" is a disposition of human remains by cremation, without formal viewing, visitation, or ceremony with the body present.

(h) <u>Funeral Goods</u> "Funeral goods" are the goods which are sold or offered for sale directly to the public for use in connection with funeral services.

(i) <u>Funeral Provider</u> A "funeral provider" is any person, partnership, or corporation that sells or offers to sell funeral goods and funeral services to the public.

(j) <u>Funeral Services</u> "Funeral services" are any services which may be used to: (1) care for and prepare deceased human bodies for burial, cremation, or other final disposition; and (2) arrange, supervise, or conduct the funeral ceremony or the final disposition of deceased human bodies.

(k) <u>Immediate Burial</u> An "immediate burial" is a disposition of human remains by burial, without formal viewing, visitation, or ceremony with the body present, except for a graveside service.

(l) <u>Memorial Service</u> A "memorial service" is a ceremony commemorating the deceased without the body present.

(m) <u>Funeral Ceremony</u> A "funeral ceremony" is a service commemorating the deceased with the body present.

(n) <u>Outer Burial Container</u> An "outer burial container" is any container which is designed for placement in the grave around the casket including, but not limited to, containers commonly known as burial vaults, grave boxes, and grave liners.

(o) <u>Person</u> A "person" is any individual, partnership, corporation, association, government or governmental subdivision or agency, or other entity.

(p) <u>Services of Funeral Director and Staff</u> The "services of funeral director and staff" are the basic services, not to be included in prices of other categories in #453.2(b)(4), that are furnished by a funeral provider in arranging any funeral, such as conducting the arrangements conference, planning the funeral, obtaining necessary permits, and placing obituary notices.

453.2 Price Disclosures
(a) <u>Unfair or Deceptive Acts or Practices</u>
In selling or offering to sell funeral goods or funeral services to the public, it is an unfair or deceptive act or practice for a funeral provider to fail to furnish accurate price information disclosing the cost to the purchaser for each of the specific funeral goods and funeral services used in connection with the disposition of deceased human bodies, including at least the price of embalming, transportation of remains, use of facilities, caskets, outer burial containers, immediate burials, or direct cremations, to persons inquiring about the purchase of funerals. Any funeral provider who complies with the preventive requirements in paragraph (b) of this section is not engaged in the unfair or deceptive acts or practices defined here.

(b) <u>Preventive Requirements</u>
To prevent these unfair or deceptive acts or practices, funeral providers must:

(1) Telephone Price Disclosure

Tell persons who ask by telephone about the funeral provider's offerings or prices any accurate information from the price lists described in paragraphs (b)(2) through (4) of this section and any other readily available information that reasonably answers the question.

(2) Casket Price List

(i) Give a printed or typewritten price list to people who inquire in person about the offerings or prices of caskets or alternative containers. The funeral provider must offer the list upon beginning discussion of, but in any event before showing, caskets. The list must contain at least the retail prices of all caskets and alternative containers offered which do not require special ordering, enough information to identify each, and the effective date for the price list. In lieu of a written list, other formats, such as notebooks, brochures, or charts may be used if they contain the same information as would the printed or typewritten list and display it in a clear and conspicuous manner. Provided, however, that funeral providers do not have to make a casket price list available if the funeral providers place on the general price list, specified in paragraph (b)(4) of this section, the information required by this paragraph.

(ii) Place on the list, however produced, the name of the funeral provider's place of business and a caption describing the list as a "Casket Price List."

(3) Outer Burial Container Price List

(i) Give a printed or typewritten price list to persons who inquire in person about outer burial container offerings or prices. The funeral provider must offer the list upon beginning discussion of, but in any event before showing, the containers. The list must contain at least the retail prices of all outer burial containers offered which do not require special ordering, enough information to identify each container, and the effective date for the prices listed. In lieu of a written list, the funeral provider may use other formats, such as notebooks, brochures, or charts, if they contain the same information as the printed or typewritten list and display it in a clear and conspicuous manner. Provided, however, that funeral providers do not have to make an outer burial container price list available if the funeral providers place on the general price list, specified in paragraph (b)(4) of this section, the information required by this paragraph.

(ii) Place on the list, however produced, the name of the funeral provider's place of business and a caption describing the list as an "Outer Burial Container Price List."

(4) General Price List
(i)(A) Give a printed or typewritten price list for retention to persons who inquire in person about the funeral goods, funeral services, or prices of funeral goods or services offered by the funeral provider. The funeral provider must give the list upon beginning discussion of any of the following:

(1) the prices of funeral goods or funeral services;

(2) the overall type of funeral service or disposition; or

(3) specific funeral goods or funeral services offered by the funeral provider.

(B) The requirement in paragraph (b)(4)(i)(A) of this section applies whether the discussion takes place in the funeral home or elsewhere. Provided, however, that when the deceased is removed for transportation to the funeral home, an in-person request at that time for authorization to embalm, required by #453.5(a)(2), does not, by itself, trigger the requirement to offer the general price list if the provider in seeking prior embalming approval discloses that embalming is not required by law except in certain special cases, if any. Any other discussion during that time about prices or the selection of funeral goods or services triggers the requirement under paragraph (b)(4)(i)(A) of this section to give consumers a general price list.

(C) The list required by paragraph (b)(4)(i)(A) of this section must contain at least the following information:

(1) The name, address, and telephone number of the funeral provider's place of business;

(2) A caption describing the list as a "General Price List"; and

(3) The effective date for the price list.

(ii) Include on the price list, in any order, the retail prices (expressed either as the flat fee, or as the price per hour, mile, or other unit of computation) and the other information specified below for at least each of the following items, if offered for sale:

(A) Forwarding of remains to another funeral home, together with a list of the services provided for any quoted price;

(B) Receiving remains from another funeral home, together with a list of the services provided for any quoted price;

(C) The price range for the direct cremations offered by the funeral provider, together with:

(1) a separate price for a direct cremation where the purchaser provides the container;

(2) separate prices for each direct cremation offered including an alternative container; and

(3) a description of the services and containers (where applicable) included in each price;

(D) The price range for the immediate burials offered by the funeral provider, together with:

(1) a separate price for an immediate burial where the purchaser provides the casket;

(2) separate prices for each immediate burial offered including a casket or alternative container; and

(3) a description of the services and container (where applicable) included in that price;

(E) Transfer of remains to the funeral home;

(F) Embalming;

(G) Other preparation of the body;

(H) Use of facilities and staff or viewing;

(I) Use of facilities and staff or funeral ceremony;

(J) Use of facilities and staff or memorial service;

(K) Use of equipment and staff for graveside service;

(L) Hearse; and

(M) Limousine.

(iii) Include on the price list, in any order, the following information:

(A) Either of the following:

(1) The price range for the caskets offered by the funeral provider, together with the statement: "A complete price list will be provided at the funeral home"; or

(2) The prices of individual caskets, disclosed in the manner specified by paragraph (b)(2)(i) of this section; and

(B) Either of the following:

(1) The price range for the outer burial containers offered by the funeral provider, together with the statement: "A complete price list will be provided at the funeral home"; or

(2) The prices of individual outer burial containers, disclosed in the manner specified by paragraph (b)(3)(i) of this section; and

(C) Either of the following:

(1) The price for the basic services of funeral director and staff, together with a list of the principal basic services provided for any quoted price and, if the charge cannot be declined by the purchaser, the statement: "This fee for our basic services will be added to the total cost of the funeral arrangements you select. (This fee is already included in our charges for direct cremations, immediate burials, and forwarding or receiving remains.)" If the charge cannot be declined by the purchaser, the quoted price shall include all charges for the recovery of unallocated funeral provider overhead, and funeral providers may include in the required disclosure the phrase "and overhead" after the word "services"; or

(2) The following statement: "Please note that a fee of (specify dollar amount) for the use of our basic services is included in the price of our caskets. This same fee shall be added to the total cost of your funeral arrangements if you provide the casket. Our services include (specify)." The fee shall include all charges for the recovery of

unallocated funeral provider overhead, and funeral providers may include in the required disclosure the phrase "and overhead" after the word "services." The statement must be placed on the general price list together with the casket price range, required by paragraph (b)(4)(iii)(A)(1) of this section, or together with the prices of individual caskets, required by (b)(4)(iii)(A)(2) of this section.

(iv) The services fee permitted by #453.2(b)(4)(iii)(C)(1) or (C)(2) is the only funeral provider fee for services, facilities, or unallocated overhead permitted by this part to be non-declinable, unless otherwise required by law.

(5) <u>Statement of Funeral Goods and Services Selected</u>

(i) Give an itemized written statement for retention to each person who arranges a funeral or other disposition of human remains, at the conclusion of the discussion of arrangements. The statement must list at least the following information:

(A) The funeral goods and funeral services selected by that person and the prices to be paid for each of them;

(B) Specifically itemized cash advance items. (These prices must be given to the extent then known or reasonably ascertainable. If the prices are not known or reasonably ascertainable, a good faith estimate shall be given and a written statement of the actual charges shall be provided before the final bill is paid); and

(C) The total cost of the goods and services selected.

(ii) The information required by this paragraph (b)(5) may be included on any contract, statement, or other document which the funeral provider would otherwise provide at the conclusion of discussion of arrangements.

(6) <u>Other Pricing Methods</u>
Funeral providers may give persons any other price information, in any other format, in addition to that required by #453.2(b)(2), (3), and (4) so long as the statement required by #453.2(b)(5) is given when required by the rule.

453.3 Misrepresentation
   (a) <u>Embalming Provisions</u>

(1) <u>Deceptive Acts or Practices</u>
In selling or offering to sell funeral goods or funeral services to the public, it is a deceptive act or practice for a funeral provider to:

(i) Represent that state or local law requires that a deceased person be embalmed when such is not the case;

(ii) Fail to disclose that embalming is not required by law except in certain special cases, if any.

(2) <u>Preventive Requirements</u>
To prevent these deceptive acts or practices, as well as the unfair or deceptive acts or practices defined in #453.4(b)(1) and 453.5(2), funeral providers must:

(i) Not represent that a deceased person is required to be embalmed for:

(A) direct cremation; ,

(B) immediate burial; or

(C) a closed casket funeral without viewing or visitation when refrigeration is available and when state or local law does not require embalming; and

(ii) Place the following disclosure on the general price list, required by #453.2(b)(4), in immediate conjunction with the price shown for embalming: "Except in certain special cases, embalming is not required by law. Embalming may be necessary, however, if you select certain funeral arrangements, such as a funeral with viewing. If you do not want embalming, you usually have the right to choose an arrangement that does not require you to pay for it, such as direct cremation or immediate burial." The phrase "except in certain special cases" need not be included in this disclosure if state or local law in the area(s) where the provider does business does not require embalming under any circumstances.

(b) Casket for Cremation Provisions

(1) Deceptive Acts or Practices
In selling or offering to sell funeral goods or funeral services to the public, it is a deceptive act or practice for a funeral provider to:

(i) Represent that state or local law requires a casket for direct cremations;

(ii) Represent that a casket is required for direct cremations.

(2) <u>Preventive Requirements</u>
To prevent these deceptive acts or practices, as well as the unfair or deceptive acts or practices defined in #453.4(a)(1), funeral providers must place the following disclosure in immediate conjunction with the price range shown for direct cremations: "If you want to arrange a direct cremation, you can use an alternative container. Alternative containers encase the body and can be made of materials like fiberboard or composition materials (with or without an outside covering). The containers we provide are (specify containers)." This disclosure only has to be placed on the general price list if the funeral provider arranges direct cremation.

(c) <u>Outer Burial Container Provisions</u>

(1) <u>Deceptive Acts or Practices</u>
In selling or offering to sell funeral goods and funeral services to the public, it is a deceptive act or practice for a funeral provider to:

(i) Represent that state or local laws or regulations, or particular cemeteries require outer burial containers when such is not the case;

(ii) Fail to disclose to persons arranging funerals that state law does not require the purchase of an outer burial container.

(2) <u>Preventive Requirements</u>
To prevent these deceptive acts or practices, funeral providers must place the following disclosure on the outer burial containers' price list, required by #453.2(b)(3)(i), or, if the prices of outer burial containers are listed on the general price list, required by #453.2(b)(4), in immediate conjunction with those prices: "In most areas of the country, state or local law does not require that you buy a container to surround the casket in the grave. However, many cemeteries require that you have such a container so that the grave will not sink in. Either a grave liner or a burial vault will satisfy these requirements." The phrase "in most areas of the country" need not be included in this disclosure if state or local law in the area(s) where the provider does business does not require a container to surround the casket in the grave.

(d) <u>General Provisions on Legal and Cemetery Requirements</u>

(1) <u>Deceptive Acts or Practices</u>
In selling or offering to sell funeral goods or funeral services to the public, it is a deceptive act or practice for funeral providers to represent that federal, state, or local laws, or particular cemeteries or crematories, require the purchase of any funeral goods or funeral services when such is not the case.

(2) <u>Preventive Requirements</u>
To prevent these deceptive acts or practices, as well as the deceptive acts or practices identified in #453.3(a)(1), #453.3(b)(1), and #453.3(c)(1), funeral pr oviders must identify and briefly describe in writing on the statement of funeral goods and services selected, required by #453.2(b)(5), any legal, cemetery, or crematory requirements which the funeral provider represents to persons as compelling the purchase of funeral goods or funeral services for the funeral which that person is arranging.

(e) <u>Provisions on Preservative and Protective Value Claims</u>
In selling or offering to sell funeral goods or funeral services to the public, it is a deceptive act or practice for a funeral provider to:

(1) Represent that funeral goods or funeral services will delay the natural decomposition of human remains for a long or indefinite time;

(2) Represent that funeral goods have protective features or will protect the body from gravesite substances when such is not the case.

(f) <u>Cash Advance Provisions</u>

(1) <u>Deceptive Acts or Practices</u>
In selling or offering to sell funeral goods or funeral services to the public, it is a deceptive act or practice for a funeral provider to:

(i) Represent that the price charged for a cash advance item is the same as the cost to the funeral provider for the item when such is not the case;

(ii) Fail to disclose to persons arranging funerals that the price being charged for the cash advance item is not the same as the cost to the funeral provider for the item when such is the case.

(2) Preventive Requirements

To prevent these deceptive acts or practices, funeral providers must place the following sentence in the itemized statement of funeral goods and services selected, in immediate conjunction with the list of itemized cash advance items required by #453.2(b)(5)(i)(B): "We charge you for our services in obtaining: (specify cash advance items)," if the funeral provider makes a charge upon, or receives and retains a rebate, commission, or trade or volume discount upon a cash advance item.

453.4 Required Purchase of Funeral Goods or Funeral Services

(a) Casket for Cremation Provisions

(1) Unfair or Deceptive Acts or Practices

In selling or offering to sell funeral goods or funeral services to the public, it is an unfair or deceptive act or practice for a funeral provider, or a crematory, to require that a casket be purchased for direct cremation.

(2) Preventive Requirement

To prevent this unfair or deceptive act or practice, funeral providers must make an alternative container available for direct cremations, if they arrange direct cremations.

(b) <u>Other Required Purchases of Funeral Goods or Funeral Services</u>

(1) <u>Unfair or Deceptive Acts or Practices</u>
In selling or offering to sell funeral goods or funeral services, it is an unfair or deceptive act or practice for a funeral provider to:

(i) Condition the furnishing of any funeral good or funeral service to a person arranging a funeral upon the purchase of any other funeral good or funeral service, except as required by law or as otherwise permitted by this part;

(ii) Charge any fee as a condition to furnishing any funeral goods or funeral services to a person arranging a funeral, other than the fees for (1) services of funeral director and staff, permitted by #453.2(b)(4)(iii)(C); (2) other funeral services and funeral goods selected by the purchaser; and (3) other funeral goods or services required to be purchased, as explained on the itemized statement in accordance with #453.3(d)(2).

(2) <u>Preventive Requirements</u>

(i) To prevent these unfair or deceptive acts or practices, funeral providers must:

(A) Place the following disclosure in the general price list, immediately above the prices required by

#453.2(b)(4)(iii): "The goods and services shown below are those we can provide to our customers. You may choose only the items you desire. If legal or other requirements mean you must buy any items you did not specifically ask for, we will explain the reason in writing on the statement we provide describing the funeral goods and services you selected." Provided, however, that if the charge for "services of funeral director and staff" cannot be declined by the purchaser, the statement shall include the sentence: "However, any funeral arrangements you select will include a charge for our basic services" between the second and third sentences of the statement specified above herein. The statement may include the phrase "and overhead" after the word "services" if the fee includes a charge for the recovery of unallocated funeral provider overhead;

(B) Place the following disclosure in the statement of funeral goods and services selected, required by #453.2(b)(5)(i): "Charges are only for those items that you selected or that we required. If we are required by law or by a cemetery or crematory to use any items, we will explain the reasons in writing below."

(ii) A funeral provider shall not violate this section by failing to comply with a request for a combination of goods or services which would be impossible, impractical, or excessively burdensome to provide.

453.5 Services Provided without Prior Approval
(a) Unfair or Deceptive Acts or Practices
In selling or offering to sell funeral goods or funeral services to the public, it is an unfair or deceptive act or

practice for any provider to embalm a deceased human body for a fee unless:

(1) State or local law or regulation requires embalming in the particular circumstances regardless of any funeral choice which the family might make; or

(2) Prior approval for embalming (expressly so described) has been obtained from a family member or other authorized person; or

(3) The funeral provider is unable to contact a family member or other authorized person after exercising due diligence, has no reason to believe the family does not want embalming performed, and obtains subsequent approval for embalming already performed (expressly so described). In seeking approval, the funeral provider must disclose that a fee will be charged if the family selects a funeral which requires embalming, such as a funeral with viewing, and that no fee will be charged if the family selects a service which does not require embalming, such as direct cremation or immediate burial.

(b) <u>Preventive Requirement</u>

To prevent these unfair or deceptive acts or practices, funeral providers must include on the itemized statement of funeral goods and services selected, required by #453.2(b)(5), the statement: "If you selected a funeral that may require embalming, such as a funeral with viewing, you may have to pay for embalming. You do not have to pay for embalming you did not approve if you selected arrangements such as a direct cremation or immediate burial. If we charged for embalming, we will explain why below."

453.6 Retention of Documents

To prevent the unfair or deceptive acts or practices specified in #453.2 and #453.3 of this r ule, funeral providers must retain and make available for inspection by Commission officials true and accurate copies of the price lists specified in #453.2(b)(2) thr ough (4), as applicable, for at least one year after the date of their last distribution to customers, and a copy of each statement of funeral goods and services selected, as required by #453.2(b)(5), for at least one year fr om the date of the arrangements conference.

453.7 Comprehension of Disclosures

To prevent the unfair or deceptive acts or practices specified in #453.2 thr ough #453.5, funeral pr oviders must make all disclosures required by those sections in a clear and conspicuous manner. Providers shall not include in the casket, outer burial container, and general price lists, required by #453.2(b)(2)-(4), any statement or information that alters or contradicts the information required by this Part to be included in those lists.

453.8 Declaration of Intent

(a) Except as otherwise provided in #453.2(a), it is a violation of this rule to engage in any unfair or deceptive acts or practices specified in this rule, or to fail to comply with any of the preventive requirements specified in this rule;

(b) The provisions of this rule are separate and severable from one another. If any provision is determined to be invalid, it is the Commission's intention that the remaining provisions shall continue in effect;

(c) This rule shall not apply to the business of insurance or to acts in the conduct thereof.

453.9 State Exemptions
If, upon application to the Commission by an appropriate state agency, the Commission determines that:

(a) There is a state requirement in effect which applies to any transaction to which this rule applies; and

(b) State requirement affords an overall level of protection to consumers which is as great as, or greater than, the protection afforded by this rule;

then the Commission's rule will not be in effect in that state to the extent specified by the Commission in its determination, for as long as the State administers and enforces effectively the state requirements.

By direction of the Commission

Donald S. Clark
Secretary

Appendix II

ABC FUNERAL HOME
100 Main Street
Yourtown, USA 12345

General Price List

These prices are effective as of (date).
The goods and services shown below are those we can
provide to our customers. You may choose only the items
you desire. However, any funeral arrangements you
select will include a charge for our basic services and
overhead. If legal or other requirements mean you must
buy any items you did not specifically ask for, we will
explain the reason in writing on the statement we provide
describing the funeral goods and services you selected.

Basic Services of Funeral Director
and Staff and Overhead .... $ _____

Our services include: conducting the arrangements
conference; planning the funeral; consulting with family
and clergy; sheltering remains; preparing and filing of
necessary notices; obtaining necessary authorizations and
permits; and coordinating with the cemetery, cremator,
or other third parties. In addition, this fee includes a
proportionate share of our basic overhead costs.

This fee for our basic services and overhead will be added to the total cost of the funeral arrangements you select. (This fee is already included in our charges for direct cremations, immediate burials, and forwarding or receiving remains.)

Embalming .... $ ———
Except in certain special cases, embalming is not required by law. Embalming may be necessary, however, if you select certain funeral arrangements, such as a funeral with viewing. If you do not want embalming, you usually have the right to choose an arrangement that does not require you to pay for it, such as direct cremation, or immediate burial.

Other Preparation of the Body .... $ ———
(list individual services and prices)

Transfer of Remains to the Funeral Home
(within __ -Mile radius) .... $ ———
beyond this radius we charge __ per mile

Use of Facilities and Staff for Viewing
at the Funeral Home .... $ ———

Use of Facilities and Staff for Funeral Ceremony
at the Funeral Home .... $ ———

Use of Facilities and Staff for Memorial Service
at the Funeral Home .... $ ———

Use of Equipment and Staff
for Graveside Service .... $ _____

Hearse .... $ _____

Limousine .... $_____

Caskets... $ _____to $_____
A complete price list will be provided at the funeral home.

Outer Burial Container .... $ _____to $_____
A complete price list will be provided at the funeral home.

Forwarding of Remains to Another
Funeral Home .... $ _____
Our charge includes: basic services of funeral director and
staff; a proportionate share of overhead costs; removal of
remains; embalming or other preparation of remains, if
relevant; and local transportation.

Receiving Remains from Another
Funeral Home .... $ _____
Our charge includes: basic services of funeral director and
staff; a proportionate share of overhead costs; care of
remains; and transportation of remains to funeral home
and to cemetery or crematory.

Direct Cremation................................. $ _____ to $ _____
Our charge for a direct cremation (without ceremony)
includes: basic services of funeral director and staff; a
proportionate share of overhead costs; removal of
remains; transportation to crematory; necessary
authorizations; and cremation, if relevant.

If you want to arrange a direct cremation, you can use an alternative container. Alternative containers encase the body and can be made of materials like fiberboard or composition materials (with or without an outside covering). The containers we provide are a fiberboard container or an unfinished wood box.

A. Direct cremation with container
provided by purchaser .... $_____

B. Direct cremation with
a fiberboard container .... $_____

C. Direct cremation with an
unfinished wood box .... $_____

Immediate Burial .... $ ____ to $_____
Our charge for an immediate burial (without ceremony) includes: basic services of funeral director and staff; a proportionate share of overhead costs; removal of remains; and local transportation to cemetery.

A. Immediate burial with casket provided
by purchaser .... $_____

B. Immediate burial with alternative
container (if offered) .... $_____

C. Immediate burial with cloth-covered
wood casket .... $_____

Appendix III

ABC FUNERAL HOME

Casket Price List

These prices are effective as of (date).

Alternative Containers:

1. Fiberboard Box .... $ _____
2. Plywood Box .... $ _____
3. Unfinished Pine Box .... $ _____

Caskets:

1. Beige cloth-covered soft-wood
with beige interior .... $ _____

2. Oak-stained soft-wood
with pleated blue crepe interior .... $ _____

3. Mahogany-finished soft-wood
with maroon crepe interior .... $ _____

4. Solid white pine
with eggshell crepe interior .... $ _____

5. Solid mahogany
with tufted rosetan velvet interior .... $_____

6. Hand finished solid cherry
with ivory velvet interior .... $_____

7. 18-gauge rose colored steel
with pleated maroon crepe interior
(available in a variety of interiors) .... $_____

8. 20-gauge bronze colored steel
with blue crepe interior .... $_____

9. Solid bronze (16-gauge) with brushed finish
white ivory velvet interior .... $_____

10. Solid copper (32 oz.) with sealer (oval glass)
and medium bronze finish
with rosetan velvet interior .... $_____

Appendix IV

ABC FUNERAL HOME

Outer Burial Container Price List

These prices are effective as of (date).

In most areas of the country, state or local law does not require that you buy a container to surround the casket in the grave. However, many cemeteries require that you have such a container so that the grave will not sink in. Either a grave liner or a burial vault satisfy these requirements.

1. Concrete Grave Liner .... $ _____

2. Acme Reinforced Concrete Vault (lined) .... $ _____

3. Acme Reinforced Concrete Vault
(stainless steel-lined) .... $ _____

4. Acme Solid Copper Vault .... $ _____

5. Acme Steel Vault (12-gauge) .... $ _____

Appendix V

ABC FUNERAL HOME

Statement of Funeral Goods and Services Selected

Charges are only for those items that you selected or that are required. If we are required by law or by a cemetery or crematory to use any items, we will explain the reasons in writing below.

Deceased:———————————————————————
Purchaser: ——————————————————————
Address:———————————————————————
Tel. No. ——————————————————————

Date of Death   Date of Arrangements
_____   _____

Basic Services of Funeral Director and Staff and Overhead.. $ _____

Embalming .... $ _____

If you selected a funeral that may require embalming, such as a funeral with viewing, you may have to pay for embalming. You do not have to pay for embalming you did not approve if you selected arrangements such as a direct cremation or immediate burial. If we charged for embalming, we will explain why below.

Other Preparation of the Body

    1. Cosmetic Work for Viewing .... $_____
    2. Washing and Disinfecting
       Unembalmed Remains .... $_____

Transfer of Remains to the
Funeral Home .... $_____

Use of Facilities and Staff
for Viewing .... $_____

Use of Facilities and Staff
for Funeral Ceremony .... $_____

Use of Facilities and Staff
for Memorial Service .... $_____

Use of Equipment and Staff
for Graveside Service .... $_____

Hearse .... $_____

Limousine .... $_____

Casket .... $_____

Outer Burial Container .... $_____

Forwarding of Remains to Another
Funeral Home .... $_____

Receiving Remains from
Another Funeral Home .... $_____

Direct Cremation .... $_____

Immediate Burial .... $_____

CASH ADVANCE ITEMS
We charge you for our services in obtaining: (specify
relevant cash advance items).

Cemetery charges .... $_____
Crematory charges .... $_____
Flowers .... $_____
Obituary notice .... $_____
Death certificate .... $_____
Music .... $_____

Total Cash Advance Items................................. $_____

TOTAL COST OF ARRANGEMENTS
(including all services, merchandise, and cash advance
items) .... $_____

If any legal, cemetery, or crematory requirements have required the purchase of any of these items listed above, we will explain the requirements below:

_____

_____

_____

Reason for Embalming:

_____

Appendix VI

Sample Body Donor Form

A REQUEST TO DONATE MY BODY
TO THE UNIVERSITY OF MINNESOTA

The University of Minnesota Bequest Program, in cooperation with other institutions of higher learning within the state, has been developed to ensure the availability of human bodies to aid in the education of Health Science Practitioners. The following information is provided to individuals who wish to request that the University consider accepting their body upon death:

THE UNIVERSITY RESERVES THE RIGHT
NOT TO ACCEPT A BODY

Under the terms of the Minnesota Anatomical Gift Act, the University of Minnesota has the right to accept or reject a body dependent upon the needs of the University and the acceptability of the body for the purposes intended, even though a form is on file prior to death. Bodies that have been autopsied, mutilated, are decomposed, overweight, die from communicable diseases, or have been organ donors (other than eye donation) are not acceptable for the purposes of anatomical study. In addition, the University of

Minnesota reserves the right to refuse a body if the condition of the body precludes adequate preparation, storage, or study.

At the Time of Death: The health care institution, physician, or the family should notify the Anatomy Bequest Program at (612) 625-1111. At that time, the staff of the Bequest Program will determine whether the body can be accepted for study, and if so, will make the necessary arrangements. If the body is not accepted, the next of kin/estate will be responsible for making final disposition arrangements.

Role of the Family at the Time of Death: If a family knows that the intentions of the deceased have changed, or if the family's needs or wishes are not served by this donation, they need not honor this form. The University should be notified that the death has occurred and that the donation will not be implemented. At that time, other arrangements for final disposition must be made, and all expenses will be the responsibility of the estate.

Funeral Services: When the family desires to have a funeral service with the body present, they should make the necessary arrangements with the funeral director of their choosing. The family must assume all financial responsibility for these arrangements. The designated funeral director should immediately contact the Anatomy Bequest Program at (612) 625-1111 to determine whether the body can be accepted for study.

Final Disposition of Remains: When the anatomical studies have been completed, which as a rule take longer than a year, three alternatives are available to the family for final disposition of the remains:

1) the University will cremate the remains and inter the cremated remains in a cemetery.

2) the University will cremate the remains and return the cremated remains to the family for final disposition of their choice. All expenses for this family-arranged final disposition will be the responsibility of the estate.

3) the University will return the entire body for burial in a cemetery. All expenses for transportation and burial will be the responsibility of the estate.

BIOGRAPHICAL INFORMATION
(necessary for death certificate)

Social Security #_____ Sex:_____ Race: _____

Date of Birth: _____ Place of Birth: _____
Marital Status: Never Married ____ Married____ Divorced ____ Widowed ____
Spouse (even if widowed):_____ (give maiden name if wife)
Your Usual Occupation: _____
(do not use retired)
Kind of Business/Industry: _____

Your <u>Highest</u> Level of Education:
1 2 3 4 5 6 7 8 9 10 11 12   1 2 3 4 5+
Elementary/Secondary   Post-Secondary
Were you ever in the U.S. Armed Forces ____Yes ____ No

Father: _____
          First   Middle   Last
Mother: _____
          First   Middle   Last

RESTRICTIONS OVER THE USE OF YOUR BODY FOR ANATOMICAL STUDY

The Anatomy Bequest Program functions to ensure the availability of bodies for teaching human anatomy. Within Minnesota, there are other institutions of higher learning that request bodies to be used in their anatomy programs. As such, bodies occasionally leave the University for study. Under the terms of this Bequest Form, you may choose any of the options listed, or you may state any restrictions you would like to apply at the time of death. The University reserves the right to refuse the bequest if we feel we cannot comply with your restrictions. Please indicate your choice below by **signing** in the space provided.

_____ No restrictions - University may do as it sees fit
_____ My body may not be used away from the University of Minnesota
_____ Other restrictions - please be specific:_____

In accordance with the Minnesota Uniform Anatomical Gift Act, if my body is accepted at the time of death, it is my desire that the University use my body to aid in the education of health science practitioners, within the restrictions (if any), that I have stipulated above.

I do understand that the University may not be able to accept my body at the time of death, in which case my next of kin will have to make other arrangements for final disposition.

_____   _____
            Signature   Date

Please Print or Type
FULL NAME: _____
            First   Middle   Last

_____
    Street Address   City   State   Zip

_____   _____
  1) Witness Signature   Date

_____   _____
  2) Witness Signature   Date

The original of this form must be on file at the University of Minnesota at the time of death. Photocopies of the original will be provided by the University, indicating the original is on file.

Index

Index

D

E

Index

Environmental Protection Agency, 121

F

Index

Inurnment. *See* Cremation, cremains, disposal of
International Cemetery and Funeral Association, 7, 100
Internet, interment on. *See* Cemeteries
Iserson, Kenneth V., 34, 81

L

Limousine. *See* Funerals, vehicles used in

M

Mausoleums
    immurement in, 44
    types of, 92-93, 97
McQueen, John, 47
Memorial gardens and parks, 91
Miller, Clarence W., 32-33
Mitford, Jessica, 121
Monuments
    comparison shopping for, 56
    definition of and descriptions, 55
    where to purchase, 55. *See also* Graves, markers for
Mortician. *See* Funeral director(s)

N

National Cemetery System, 93-95
National Concrete Burial Vault Association, 123
National Funeral Directors Association, 7, 29, 122, 135,
       172. *See also Director, The*
Newsweek, predicts future changes, 145

O

Obituaries, 59
Occupational Safety and Health Administration, 121
Outer Burial Container Price List. *See* FTC Funeral
       Industry Practices Rule
Overton, Bruce, 174

Index

Trust funds. *See* Prearrangements

U

Undertaker. *See* Funeral director(s)
United States Department of Veterans Affairs, 95

V

Vaults
    as grave liners, 48-49
    costs of, 54
    protection offered by, 31-32
    selection of, 182
    styles of, 48-49
Veterans, burials. *See* United States Department of
    Veterans Affairs

W

Wall Street Journal
    Funeral Rule Offenders Program, 135
    describes a funeral party, 143
Waltrip, Robert L., 140